Innovative Technology Based Interventions for Psychological Treatment of Common Mental Disorders

Innovative Technology Based Interventions for Psychological Treatment of Common Mental Disorders

Editors

Tara Donker
Annet Kleiboer

MDPI • Basel • Beijing • Wuhan • Barcelona • Belgrade • Manchester • Tokyo • Cluj • Tianjin

Editors
Tara Donker
Vrije Universiteit Amsterdam and
Amsterdam Public Health Research
Institute Amsterdam
The Netherlands

Annet Kleiboer
Vrije Universiteit Amsterdam and
Amsterdam Public Health Research
Institute Amsterdam
The Netherlands

Editorial Office
MDPI
St. Alban-Anlage 66
4052 Basel, Switzerland

This is a reprint of articles from the Special Issue published online in the open access journal *Journal of Clinical Medicine* (ISSN 2077-0383) (available at: https://www.mdpi.com/journal/jcm/special_issues/Innovative_Technology_Mental_Disorders).

For citation purposes, cite each article independently as indicated on the article page online and as indicated below:

LastName, A.A.; LastName, B.B.; LastName, C.C. Article Title. *Journal Name* **Year**, *Volume Number*, Page Range.

ISBN 978-3-03943-735-1 (Hbk)
ISBN 978-3-03943-736-8 (PDF)

Contents

About the Editors vii

Tara Donker and Annet Kleiboer
Innovative Technology Based Interventions for Psychological Treatment of Common Mental Disorders
Reprinted from: *J. Clin. Med.* **2020**, *9*, 3075, doi:10.3390/jcm9103075 1

Desirée Colombo, Javier Fernández-Álvarez, Andrea Patané, Michelle Semonella, Marta Kwiatkowska, Azucena García-Palacios, Pietro Cipresso, Giuseppe Riva and Cristina Botella
Current State and Future Directions of Technology-Based Ecological Momentary Assessment and Intervention for Major Depressive Disorder: A Systematic Review
Reprinted from: *J. Clin. Med.* **2019**, *8*, 465, doi:10.3390/jcm8040465 5

Claire R. van Genugten, Josien Schuurmans, Femke Lamers, Harriëtte Riese, Brenda W. J. H. Penninx, Robert A. Schoevers, Heleen M. Riper and Johannes H. Smit
Experienced Burden of and Adherence to Smartphone-Based Ecological Momentary Assessment in Persons with Affective Disorders
Reprinted from: *J. Clin. Med.* **2020**, *9*, 322, doi:10.3390/jcm9020322 31

Nickolai Titov, Heather D. Hadjistavropoulos, Olav Nielssen, David C. Mohr, Gerhard Andersson and Blake F. Dear
From Research to Practice: Ten Lessons in Delivering Digital Mental Health Services
Reprinted from: *J. Clin. Med.* **2019**, *8*, 1239, doi:10.3390/jcm8081239 45

Mayke Mol, Claire van Genugten, Els Dozeman, Digna J. F. van Schaik, Stasja Draisma, Heleen Riper and Jan H. Smit
Why Uptake of Blended Internet-Based Interventions for Depression Is Challenging: A Qualitative Study on Therapists' Perspectives
Reprinted from: *J. Clin. Med.* **2020**, *9*, 91, doi:10.3390/jcm9010091 59

Lisa Kooistra, Jeroen Ruwaard, Jenneke Wiersma, Patricia van Oppen and Heleen Riper
Working Alliance in Blended Versus Face-to-Face Cognitive Behavioral Treatment for Patients with Depression in Specialized Mental Health Care
Reprinted from: *J. Clin. Med.* **2020**, *9*, 347, doi:10.3390/jcm9020347 81

Nadine Friedl, Tobias Krieger, Karine Chevreul, Jean Baptiste Hazo, Jérôme Holtzmann, Mark Hoogendoorn, Annet Kleiboer, Kim Mathiasen, Antoine Urech, Heleen Riper and Thomas Berger
Using the Personalized Advantage Index for Individual Treatment Allocation to Blended Treatment or Treatment as Usual for Depression in Secondary Care
Reprinted from: *J. Clin. Med.* **2020**, *9*, 490, doi:10.3390/jcm9020490 97

Christian Moser, Rahel Bachem, Thomas Berger and Andreas Maercker
ZIEL: Internet-Based Self-Help for Adjustment Problems: Results of a Randomized Controlled Trial
Reprinted from: *J. Clin. Med.* **2019**, *8*, 1655, doi:10.3390/jcm8101655 113

Tara Donker, Chris van Klaveren, Ilja Cornelisz, Robin N. Kok and Jean-Louis van Gelder
Analysis of Usage Data from a Self-Guided App-Based Virtual Reality Cognitive Behavior Therapy for Acrophobia: A Randomized Controlled Trial
Reprinted from: *J. Clin. Med.* **2020**, *9*, 1614, doi:10.3390/jcm9061614 129

About the Editors

Tara Donker is Associate Professor at the Department of Clinical Psychology, Vrije Universiteit Amsterdam, the Netherlands, and Senior Researcher at Albert-Ludwig University of Freiburg, Germany. She is also a licensed health care psychologist and has a registration in cognitive behavior therapy (VGCt). Her research focuses on early intervention and prevention of depression, anxiety, and suicide based on innovative technologies such as virtual reality and mobile apps. Her main goal is to make mental health care more accessible and scalable.

Annet Kleiboer is Associate Professor at the Department of Clinical, Neuro, and Developmental Psychology at the Vrije Universiteit Amsterdam, the Netherlands. Her research and teaching are focused on developing and testing the effects of low-intensity interventions for the prevention and treatment of common mental disorders and, in particular, how digital technologies can optimize these treatments.

Journal of
Clinical Medicine

MDPI

Editorial

Innovative Technology Based Interventions for Psychological Treatment of Common Mental Disorders

Tara Donker [1,2,3,*] and Annet Kleiboer [1,2]

1 Department of Clinical, Neuro and Developmental Psychology, Section Clinical Psychology, Vrije Universiteit Amsterdam, Van der Boechorststraat 1, 1081 BT Amsterdam, The Netherlands; a.m.kleiboer@vu.nl

2 Amsterdam Public Health Research Institute Amsterdam, Van der Boechorststraat 7, 1081 BT Amsterdam, The Netherlands

3 Department of Psychology, Laboratory of Biological and Personality Psychology, Albert Ludwigs-University of Freiburg, Peter-Kaplan Meierstrasse 8, 79104 Freiburg im Breisgau, Germany

* Correspondence: t.donker@vu.nl

Received: 15 September 2020; Accepted: 16 September 2020; Published: 24 September 2020

The present Special Issue of *Journal of Clinical Medicine* includes a series of important papers that aim to further the evidence base of innovative technological advances in the screening and treatment of mental health, and to further our understanding of their implications for mental health care.

The article by Colombo et al. [1] provides a systematic review of technology-based ecological momentary assessment (EMA) and ecological momentary intervention (EMI) for Major Depressive Disorder (MDD). EMA refers to assessments that take place in the environment of the participant close to the time of the experience. EMI refers to interventions in the environment of the participants close to the time of the experience. Their systematic review identified 32 studies using EMA for the assessment of MDD and eight studies targeting EMI. The authors concluded that the widespread adoption of EMA for the investigation of MDD has led to novel insights into different aspects of the disease, including emotion reactivity, cortisol patterns and daily rumination. This review found only four EMIs for depression, two of which were tested in a randomized controlled trial (RCT). Although results seem encouraging, more high-quality EMI trials are needed as well as improving individual tailoring and engagement of EMAs and EMIs. Furthermore, the gap between research and clinical practice is quite wide, as evidenced by the low number of studies in clinical settings. Elaborating on this topic, the paper of Genugten et al. [2] investigated the experienced burden of and adherence to EMA in persons with current affective disorders; remitted persons; and healthy controls. Results demonstrated that EMAs are slightly more burdensome to persons with affective disorders but that that does not impact adherence. They concluded that EMA is feasible to apply to persons with affective disorders.

The paper by Titov et al. [3] provides 10 lessons that the authors have learned while establishing and delivering internet-delivered interventions through Digital Mental Health Services (DMHS) as part of routine care. With their findings they anticipated that these lessons would help those launching similar clinics. The authors learned that DMHS can improve access to care for those who really need care, that DMHS deliver more than treatment services (namely, information and assessment services) and that DMHS are used by a broad-cross-section of the population. Furthermore, it is important that robust systems for therapist training are in place and supervision of therapists is essential. Additionally, specialist skills to operate DMHS are required (e.g., developing expertise in the evaluation of risk via telephone or online communication). The authors further learned about the importance of external-facing activities to overcome challenges of integrating DMHS within health systems (e.g., the challenging complexity of health systems and their resistance to change) and that DMHS can inform future mental health policy to help improve the broader mental health system by presenting data drawn from a broad cross section of the community. Despite the challenges, the authors are highly optimistic about the potential of DMHS to reduce the global burden of the high prevalence of mental health disorders. Elaborating on dissemination of Internet-delivered treatment in routine care, the paper of Mol et al. [4] describes a qualitative study targeting therapists' perspectives of blended Internet-delivered interventions, specifically, cognitive behavioural therapy (CBT). In blended Internet-delivered interventions, face-to-face treatment with a therapist was combined with online therapy. The results demonstrated that therapists were positive about blended CBT (bCBT) and that high uptake was expected but that therapists did not experience time-savings—rather the opposite. In line with Titov et al. [3], they also reported that training therapists is very important to overcome barriers of Internet-delivered CBT uptake. Challenges that were identified included technical issues and a difficulty integrating bCBT in daily life. bCBT was also the focus of research in the paper by Kooistra et al. [5]. In this paper, results from an RCT in which the working alliance in bCBT vs. face-to-face CBT for depression in specialized mental health were reported. The authors demonstrated that working alliance ratings were high in both groups by both patients and therapists. This means that replacing a proportion of the face-to-face sessions with online sessions and online therapist feedback did not have a negative effect on working alliance and treatment effect. The authors noted that in the face-to-face CBT condition but not in bCBT, lower depression scores were associated with higher alliance ratings. They concluded that the online component of bCBT may have led patients to evaluate the working alliance differently from patients receiving face-to-face CBT only.

In the paper by Friedl et al. [6], the authors investigated what the most important predictors are in determining optimal treatment allocation to treatment as usual or blended treatment. Furthermore, they investigated if model-determined treatment allocation using this predictive information and the personalized advantage index (PAI) approach would result in better outcomes. Using data from an RCT comparing efficacy of treatment as usual and blended treatment in depressive outpatients, they demonstrated that two prognostic predictors, namely, pre-treatment symptomatology and treatment expectancy, influence optimal treatment allocation but that this needs to be tested empirically. Furthermore, the results also showed an advantage of model-determined treatment allocation. One-third of the patients had a PAI larger than 5, meaning they would have improved significantly if they had received their "optimal" treatment.

In the paper of Moser et al. [7], the authors investigated an Internet-delivered self-help treatment targeting adjustment problems. The authors used an RCT design among n = 98 participants that were randomly assigned to care as usual (CAU) or CAU plus the online intervention. Results demonstrated a comparable reduction of symptom burden in both groups, while significantly fewer depressive symptoms and significantly higher quality of life were demonstrated in the experimental group. The usability of the intervention was rated above average. These results suggest that their intervention "Back to your own life" (German acronym: ZIEL), may contribute to the treatment of Adjustment Disorder by means of a scalable low-barrier approach.

Finally, in the paper by Donker et al. [8], user engagement with a self-guided app-based virtual reality (VR) CBT for acrophobia symptoms was examined. Results demonstrated that the majority of participants continued to finish all VR levels and that self-reported fear consistently decreased between the start and finish of level. The authors suggest that it might be more beneficial to play one level for a longer time period instead of practicing many VR levels. Most participants progressed effectively to the highest self-exposure level, despite the absence of a therapist.

All in all, results from the papers in this Special Issue show that technological interventions can increase the scalability and dissemination of treatment for patients in need, and that they do not affect treatment outcome or working alliance, although there are many barriers to overcome, such as training of therapists, technical problems and complex health care systems. More research is needed to investigate such interventions in naturalistic settings.

Funding: This research received no external funding.

Conflicts of Interest: The authors declare no conflict of interest.

References

1. Colombo, D.; Fernandez-Alvarez, J.; Patane, A.; Semonella, M.; Kiwatkowska, M.; Garcia-Palacios, A.; Cipresso, P.; Riva, G.; Botella, C. Current state and future directions of technology-based ecological momentary assessment and intervention for major depressive disorder: A systematic review. *J. Clin. Med.* **2019**, *8*, 465.
2. van Genugten, C.; Schuurmans, J.; Lamers, F.; Riese, H.; Penninx, B.W.J.H.; Schoevers, R.A.; Riper, H.M.; Smit, J.H. Experieced burden of and adherence to smartphone-based ecological momentary assessment in persons with affective disorders. *J. Clin. Med.* **2020**, *9*, 322.
3. Titov, N.; Hadjistavropoulos, H.D.; Nielssen, O.; Mohr, D.C.; Andersson, G.; Dear, B.F. From research to practice: Ten lessons in delivering digital mental health services. *J. Clin. Med.* **2019**, *8*, 1239. [CrossRef] [PubMed]
4. Mol, M.; van Genugten, C.; Dozeman, E.; van Schaik, D.J.F.; Draisma, S.; Riper, H.; Smit, J.H. Why uptake of blended internet-based interventions for depression is challenging: A qualitative study on therapists perspectives. *J. Clin. Med.* **2020**, *9*, 91. [CrossRef] [PubMed]
5. Kooistra, L.; Ruwaard, J.; Wiersma, J.; van Oppen, P.; Riper, H. Working alliance in blended versus face-to-face cognitive behavioral treatment for patients with depression in specialized mental health care. *J. Clin. Med.* **2020**, *9*, 347. [CrossRef] [PubMed]
6. Friedl, N.; Krieger, T.; Chevreul, K.; Hazo, J.B.; Holtzmann, J.; Hoogendoorn, M.; Kleiboer, A.; Mathiasen, K.; Urech, A.; Riper, H.; et al. Using the personalized advantage index for individual treatment allocation to blended treatment or treatment as usual for depression in secondary care. *J. Clin. Med.* **2020**, *9*, 490.
7. Moser, C.; Bachem, R.; Berger, T.; Maercker, A. ZIEL: Internet-based self-help for adjustment problems: Results of a randomized-controlled trial. *J. Clin. Med.* **2019**, *8*, 1655. [CrossRef]
8. Donker, T.; van Klaveren, C.; Cornelisz, I.; Kok, R.N.; van Gelder, J.L. Analysis of usage data from a self-guided app-based virtual reality cognitive behavior therapy for acrophobia: A randomized controlled trial. *J. Clin. Med.* **2020**, *9*, 1614. [CrossRef] [PubMed]

Journal of
Clinical Medicine

MDPI

Review

Current State and Future Directions of Technology-Based Ecological Momentary Assessment and Intervention for Major Depressive Disorder: A Systematic Review

Desirée Colombo [1,*], Javier Fernández-Álvarez [2], Andrea Patané [3], Michelle Semonella [4], Marta Kwiatkowska [3], Azucena García-Palacios [1,5], Pietro Cipresso [2,4], Giuseppe Riva [2,4] and Cristina Botella [1,5]

1 Department of Basic Psychology, Clinic and Psychobiology, Universitat Jaume I, Av. Sos Baynat, s/n, 12071 Castellón, Spain; azucena@uji.es (A.G.-P.); botella@uji.es (C.B.)
2 Department of Psychology, Università Cattolica del Sacro Cuore, Largo Gemelli, 1, 20100 Milan, Italy; javier.fernandezkirszman@unicatt.it (J.F.-Á.); pietro.cipresso@unicatt.it (P.C.); giuseppe.riva@unicatt.it (G.R.)
3 Department of Computer Science, University of Oxford, Wolfson Building, Parks Rd, Oxford OX1 3QD, UK; andrea.patane@cs.ox.ac.uk (A.P.); marta.kwiatkowska@cs.ox.ac.uk (M.K.)
4 Applied Technology for Neuro-Psychology Lab, IRCCS Istituto Auxologico Italiano, 20149 Milan, Italy; semonellamichelle@gmail.com
5 CIBER Fisiopatología Obesidad y Nutrición (CIBERobn), Instituto Salud Carlos III, 28029 Madrid, Spain
* Correspondence: dcolombo@uji.es; Tel.: +34-964-387-644

Received: 6 March 2019; Accepted: 1 April 2019; Published: 5 April 2019

Abstract: Ecological momentary assessment (EMA) and ecological momentary intervention (EMI) are alternative approaches to retrospective self-reports and face-to-face treatments, and they make it possible to repeatedly assess patients in naturalistic settings and extend psychological support into real life. The increase in smartphone applications and the availability of low-cost wearable biosensors have further improved the potential of EMA and EMI, which, however, have not yet been applied in clinical practice. Here, we conducted a systematic review, using the Preferred Reporting Items for Systematic Reviews and Meta-Analyses (PRISMA) guidelines, to explore the state of the art of technology-based EMA and EMI for major depressive disorder (MDD). A total of 33 articles were included (EMA = 26; EMI = 7). First, we provide a detailed analysis of the included studies from technical (sampling methods, duration, prompts), clinical (fields of application, adherence rates, dropouts, intervention effectiveness), and technological (adopted devices) perspectives. Then, we identify the advantages of using information and communications technologies (ICTs) to extend the potential of these approaches to the understanding, assessment, and intervention in depression. Furthermore, we point out the relevant issues that still need to be addressed within this field, and we discuss how EMA and EMI could benefit from the use of sensors and biosensors, along with recent advances in machine learning for affective modelling.

Keywords: major depressive disorder; ecological momentary assessment; ecological momentary intervention

1. Introduction

Major depressive disorder (MDD) is a common debilitating psychiatric disease characterized by mood disturbances, loss of interest and pleasure in daily activities, disturbed appetite and sleep, loss of energy, and psychomotor retardation or agitation. According to the World Health Organization, depression is one of the leading causes of disease and disability in the world, annually affecting 4.4%

of the general adult population [1]. In addition to producing high costs for the public health system, depression seriously impairs patients' functioning, leading to increased mortality, high suicide rates, exacerbated medical conditions, and high consumption of alcohol and illegal drugs [2–5].

As a result of the increased availability of smartphones and portable and wearable devices, a growing body of research has begun to explore new digital technologies as potential tools to foster assessments and interventions in clinical practice. More specifically, technology-based ecological momentary assessment (EMA) and ecological momentary intervention (EMI) have been proposed as alternative strategies to assess patients ecologically in naturalistic settings and deliver psychological support in daily life.

1.1. Ecological Momentary Assessment

Traditional clinical assessments are based on retrospective self-reports in which patients are asked to summarize their symptoms and affective experiences over the past few weeks. Nevertheless, increasing evidence shows that these tools are not able to capture MDD dynamics, such as symptom fluctuations or mood shifts over time [6,7]. Likewise, self-reports are affected by recall bias. In other words, depressed patients have been found to alter the content of past experiences when asked to retrieve them retrospectively [8,9], judging symptoms as more severe [10] or increasing the elaboration of negative information [11].

EMA emerged as an alternative assessment strategy to better grasp affective and behavioural dynamics in daily life [12–14]. Not surprisingly, a growing body of research has applied this approach to exploring mood disorders [15,16]. On the one hand, the term "ecological" refers to the environment where the data are collected. Behaviours, thoughts, and affect are repeatedly written down in real-world contexts. On the other hand, the term "momentary" refers to the focus of the assessment, i.e., close in time to the experience. The first studies to use this approach adopted paper-and-pencil daily diaries, but the discomfort, low compliance, and low experimental control over backfilling made them not very efficacious [14]. The exponential progress of information and communication technologies (ICTs) and the increasing availability of smartphones offered novel opportunities to ecologically assess patients. On the one hand, mobile technologies allow the shortcomings of traditional diaries to be overcome by eliminating the need for manual data entry and by increasing control on backfilling, thus obtaining more accurate data. On the other hand, all the necessary processes can be integrated in one tool, for instance, a smartphone, thus decreasing intrusiveness and increasing users' comfort, and providing a more engaging and dynamic experience. During the day, indeed, patients are automatically prompted by the device to fill in self-reports that are subsequently stored and safely sent to clinicians and/or researchers. More recently, the potential of EMA was extended due to the integration of self-reports with data gathered from embedded sensors and wearable biosensors, hence allowing for a multimodal approach. Unobtrusive wearable biosensors can continuously monitor physiological parameters throughout the day with high precision [17], whereas smartphone embedded sensors make it possible to indirectly collect data about patients' behaviours and habits, such as their social media use, physical activity, or social interactions [18,19]. Overall, the integration of these tools has the potential to revolutionize traditional assessments, leading to the exploration of new facets of MDD obtained in daily life contexts that are often difficult to capture in laboratory settings.

1.2. Ecological Momentary Intervention

According to statistics, 70% of people suffering from mental disorders do not receive adequate psychological treatment or reach complete clinical remission [20]. Affordances of technological developments, as Kazdin and Blase suggested, may facilitate new solutions for disseminating evidence-based psychotherapy [21].

The same "ecological" and "momentary" principles have been applied to the development of innovative interventions (EMI) [22] that go beyond traditional clinical settings and extend the delivery of psychological support into real life [23]. EMI has the advantage of providing psychological support directly on hand-held mobile technologies during the flow of daily experiences, in real-time settings, and at specific time points in the day, without the need for face-to-face meetings with a clinician [24]. EMIs can be delivered both as stand-alone treatments or in combination with other treatments. Moreover, similarly to EMAs, the use of data gathered from biosensors and embedded sensors along with machine learning techniques can increase the customization of the proposed interventions [16,25].

1.3. Objectives

Recent studies have confirmed the feasibility of mobile health (mHealth) applications and patients' interest in and adherence to these technologies, suggesting the great potential of this approach in the clinical field [23,26]. Nevertheless, no systematic review has explored technology-based EMA and EMI for MDD to date. Although two reviews focused on EMAs for mood disorders [15,16], most of the included studies were based on paper-and-pencil daily diaries, and the target population included adults and adolescents with bipolar disorder (BD) and borderline personality disorder (BPD).

Coinciding with our field of interest, the aim of this systematic review is to provide an overview of the state of the art of technology-based EMA and EMI for MDD from both a clinical and technological point of view. Our final objective is to show how and why clinical practice could benefit from the use of these approaches. In doing so, we will describe the potential of new technologies in this field, and we will discuss how EMAs and EMIs could be performed with sensors and biosensors along with recent advances in machine learning for affective modelling.

2. Methods

Preferred Reporting Items for Systematic Reviews and Meta-Analyses (PRISMA) criteria [27] were followed. For the systematic review protocol, see [28].

2.1. Search Strategy

To collect relevant publications, a computer-based search was performed (March 2019). We searched in two high-order databases, PubMed and Web of Science (Web of Knowledge), using the following string: ((EMA) OR ("ecological momentary assessment") OR (EMI) OR ("mobile health") OR (mhealth) OR (smartphone) OR ("ecological momentary intervention") OR (ESM) OR ("experience sampling method") OR ("ambulatory assessment") OR ("personal digital assistant") OR ("ambulatory monitoring") OR ("real time data capture") OR ("real time monitoring") OR ("real time interventions") OR ("electronic diary") OR ("repeated observations") OR ("diary data") OR ("time series")) AND (("affective disorder") OR ("mood disorder") OR (depress*) OR (depression) OR (MDD) OR ("major depressive disorder") OR ("major depression") OR ("unipolar depression") OR ("affective symptoms").

This search produced a total of 4993 articles. After eliminating duplicate papers, we made a first selection by reading titles and abstracts, and 401 articles were retrieved. We finally selected publications by applying the selection criteria described in the following paragraph, obtaining 40 papers.

Three individual researchers (D.C., J.F.-Á., and M.S.) performed the search for publications in the English language. More details are provided in Table 1 and in the flow diagram (Figure 1), in order to make this search replicable in the future.

Table 1. Detailed search strategy.

Process	Results
PubMed/Medline	2758
Web of Science	2235
Total	4993
Not duplicated	3613
Excluded (after reading title and abstract)	3212
Retrieved	401
Excluded (after applying inclusion criteria)	361
Excluded (missing experimental data)	0
Final included articles	40

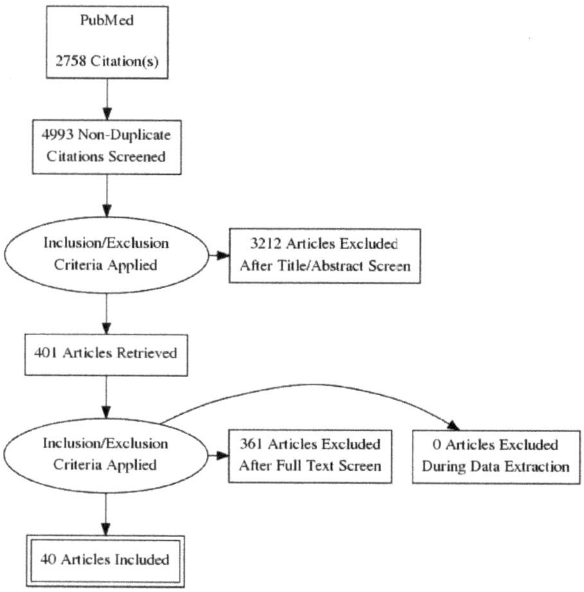

Figure 1. PRISMA (Preferred Reporting Items for Systematic Reviews and Meta-Analyses) flow diagram.

2.2. Selection Criteria

We included all studies involving a sample of adults with a primary (both current or past) diagnosis of MDD, using recognised diagnostic criteria (Diagnostic and Statistical Manual of Mental Disorders—DSM; International Classification of Disease—ICD). We excluded non-English papers and studies that did not meet the inclusion criteria. We also excluded articles that did not have full-text available, and the following types of manuscripts: Conference papers, reviews and systematic reviews, metanalyses, meeting abstracts, notes, case reports, letters to the editor, editor's notes, extended abstracts, proceedings, patents, editorials, and other editorial materials. We tried to contact the corresponding authors, when necessary, to obtain missing or supplementary data.

Ecological momentary assessment: We included studies that adopted an ecological momentary assessment by means of hand-held technologies (such as smartphones, personal digital assistants, or hand-held computers) for the collection of daily self-reports, thus excluding studies that used paper-and-pencil diaries. Additionally, we included studies that integrated daily self-reports with data supplied by sensors and biosensors.

Ecological momentary interventions: We included EMIs that were provided to patients through hand-held technologies. We selected studies in which the proposed EMI was either a stand-alone intervention or combined with other types of treatment. We also included EMI that collected data from wearable biosensors or device-embedded sensors. Because providing continuous feedback to patients has been shown to be a valuable therapeutic procedure [29], we also included studies that adopted EMA-based feedback as a therapeutic tool for clinically depressed patients.

2.3. Quality Assessment and Data Abstraction

To control for the risk of bias, PRISMA recommendations for systematic literature analysis were followed. Studies were independently selected by three different authors (D.C., M.S., and J.F.-Á.), who first analysed titles and abstracts and subsequently selected the full papers that met the inclusion criteria, resolving disagreements through consensus. For what concerns the EMA included studies, the main aim was to provide a perspective of clinical, technical, and technological issues related to this approach: In other words, we were interested in EMA as a clinical and experimental tool to be used in the psychological field, regardless of the study design or variables of outcome (Colombo et al., 2018). No risk of bias assessment was therefore performed. Differently, risk of bias of EMI studies was assessed by two independent reviewers (D.C and J.F.-Á.). As both randomized and non-randomized controlled trials were included, quality assessment was assessed with the Downs and Black quality index [30].

The data extracted from each study were as follows: Author(s), sample(s), variable(s), device(s), sensor(s), duration, prompt(s) per day, sampling schema, primary outcome(s) for the selected studies on EMA (Table 2); and author(s), name of the intervention, sample(s), content of the intervention, duration, device(s), sensor(s), and primary outcome(s) for the studies proposing an EMI (Table 3).

3. Results

3.1. Ecological Momentary Assessment in MDD

After applying the inclusion criteria, 32 studies were retrieved that investigated and assessed MDD through a technology-based EMA.

A synthesis of the results is provided in Table 2.

3.1.1. Electronic Devices and Use of Sensors

Most of the selected studies administered daily self-reports either through a personal digital assistant (PDA) or a smartphone. Only three studies adopted different technological solutions that allowed them to collect both self-reports and data gathered from sensors and biosensors. Conrad et al. [31] used the LifeShirt System (Vivometrics, Inc., Ventura, CA, USA), a comfortable garment with integrated biosensors that can continuously monitor various cardiopulmonary parameters, including heart rate (HR), respiration, and posture. With an embedded hand-held computer, patients can also complete self-reports following daily beep signals. In another study, Kim and colleagues adopted ECOLOG [32], a watch-type computer characterized by an 8-direction joystick and an integrated actimetry sensor. Via a beep signal, the wristwatch prompts patients to complete momentary assessments directly on the watch screen. Similarly, a compact wrist–worn electronic diary was used by Littlewood et al. to collect both self-reports and sleep/wake cycles with an embedded actimetry sensor [33].

Although a growing number of studies analyse data from embedded-sensors and biosensors in research on mental health disorders [34], their use in association with EMA has been low in the field of MDD. Among our selected studies, only seven of the 32 studies collected physiological measures in addition to self-reports. Conrad and colleagues collected cardiac and respiratory measures as indices of vagal activity, along with physical activity measured through an embedded actimetry sensor [31], whereas Ottaviani and colleagues collected ambulatory HR [35]. The remaining five articles investigated the association of depressive symptoms with sleep/wake cycles [32,33,36] and physical activity [37,38] using actimetry sensors.

Table 2. More detailed information about the selected Ecological Momentary Assessment studies.

	Authors	Sample	Variables	Device(s)	Duration	Prompts Per Day	Sampling Schema	Compliance	Sensor(s)	Primary Outcome(s)
Recall bias	[8]	MDD (n = 26), and HCG (n = 25)	Affect	Palm Tungsten E2	7 days	8	Semi-randomized	89%	No	Both depressed and non-depressed participants overestimate the retrospective recall of PA and NA. Depressed patients are more inaccurate in recalling NA.
	[26]	MDD (n = 13)	Randomized items from PHQ-9 questionnaire	"Mindful Moods" mobile application	29/30 days	3	Randomized	78%	No	Even if strongly correlated, the PHQ-9 scores collected through the mobile application are significantly higher than those obtained though the retrospective paper-and-pencil PHQ-9.
Symptoms monitoring	[39]	MDD (n = 20), and BD (n = 21)	Affect; stressors; behaviours; environment; social context	PDA	3 days	5	Fixed sampling scheme	85.7%	No	High rates of acceptance and compliance are observed among both samples. Participants show a practice effect, i.e., faster responses over the course of the study.
	[40]	MDD (n = 26)	Depressive and anxiety symptoms	Palm Treo 650 Smartphone (Mental Health Telemetry mobile application)	14 days	1	Selected by the patient	Not specified	No	Self-reported ratings of improvement at day 7 predict response to the treatment.
	[41]	MDD (n = 59)	Symptoms, sleep patterns, cognitive functioning	iHOPE smartphone application	8 weeks	2 (symptoms) 1 (sleep duration and quality)	Not specified	Not specified	No	Baseline depression scores evaluated with HAM-D are associated with scores of PHQ-9, VAS for depression and anxiety symptoms collected with the application.
Cortisol	[42]	MDD (n = 32), mD (n = 18), and HCG (n = 50)	Daily activities (frequency, social contacts); cortisol	Palm Pilot M100	4 days (over a maximum period of 7 days)	4 (saliva samples) 1 (self-report)	Fixed sampling scheme	Not specified	No	In the control sample, daily activities are negatively associated with cortisol levels. This association is not observed in depressed patients.
	[43]	MDD (n = 37), and HCG (n = 36)	Sleep patterns; social contacts; cortisol	Palm Pilot M100	3 non-consecutive days (over a maximum period of 7 days)	3 (saliva samples) 1 (self-report)	Fixed sampling scheme	93%	No	Depressed patients show lower cortisol awakening response, lower sleep quality, and more negative social interactions.
	[31]	MDD (n = 46) and HCG (n = 19)	Physiological indices (HR, respiration, accelerometer, cortisol); mood	LifeShirt System, with an integrated hand-held computer	1 day	6 (self-reports) 5 (saliva samples)	Fixed sampling scheme	91%	LifeShirt System (HR, respiration, actigraphy)	Cortisol level and HRV do not differ between the two groups. Interestingly, NA is negatively correlated with HRV only in the control sample.
	[44]	Remitted MDD (n = 31) and HCG (n = 32)	Mood; ruminative self-focus; stressful events; cortisol	Palm Tungsten E2	2 consecutive days	10	Semi-randomized	94%	No	Rumination and low mood are associated with increased activation of the HPAA. In remitted patients, HPAA is less responsive to subtle emotional events.
	[36]	MDD (n = 15), and HCG (n = 15)	Affect; cognition; daily activities; cortisol	PsyMate	30 days	3	Fixed sampling scheme	92.5%	ActiCal (Respironics, Bend, OR, USA)	Compared to healthy participants, depressed patients report higher cortisol levels, higher α-amylase levels, and a greater ratio of α-amylase over cortisol. This latter association, however, disappears when correction for lifestyle factors is applied.
	[45]	MDD (n = 15), and HCG (n = 15)	Affect; cortisol	PsyMate	30 days	3	Fixed sampling scheme	92.5%	No	PA and NA are bidirectionally associated with cortisol levels. Nevertheless, the direction, sign, and timing of this association show great variability among subjects.

Table 2. *Cont.*

	Authors	Sample	Variables	Device(s)	Duration	Prompts Per Day	Sampling Schema	Compliance	Sensor(s)	Primary Outcome(s)
Sleep patterns	[46]	MDD (n = 35), mD (n = 25), and HCG (n = 36)	Positive and negative affects	PDA	3 days	10	Semi-randomized	65%	No	Sleep quality predicts lower PA, but not NA. Low PA is associated with poor subjective sleep quality and self-reported daily dysfunction.
	[47]	MDD and mD (n = 60), and HCG (n = 35)	Positive and negative affects; events appraisal	Palm Pilot Zire 22	3 days	10	Semi-randomized	65%	No	In the non-clinical sample, sleep disturbances are associated with enhanced NA in response to negative events. Considering depressed patients, sleep disturbances negatively influence the emotional reactivity to both neutral and negative events.
	[48]	MDD (n = 27), and HCG (n = 27)	PA and NA, sleep quality; tiredness; rumination	PsyMate	30 days	3	Fixed sampling scheme	96%	No	Sleep quality directly influences PA and NA experienced during the following day, but not vice versa. Tiredness is a mediator.
	[49]	MDD (n = 14) and HCG (n = 15)	PA; NA; fatigue; sleep; activities; cognition; melatonin	PsyMate	30 days	3	Fixed sampling scheme	93%	No	Melatonin is associated with changes in affect and fatigue. However, changes in affect and fatigue are also predictors of melatonin levels. Individuals that do not show this association report higher depression severity and worse sleep quality.
	[38]	MDD (n = 27), and HCG (n = 27)	Sleep patterns	PsyMate	30 days	3	Fixed sampling scheme	96%	ActiCal (Respironics, Bend, OR, USA)	Sleep duration affects next-day physical activity. Depression does not moderate this association.
	[33]	MDD (n = 51)	Sleep patterns and quality; suicide ideation; entrapment perception	PRO-Diary actigraph watch (CamNtech)	7 days	6	Semi-randomized	89%	Accelerometer	Poor sleep quality, both objectively and subjectively evaluated, is associated with higher next-day suicide ideations. Suicide ideation does not influence sleep patterns and quality.
Physical activity	[50]	MDD (n = 53), and HCG (n = 53)	Physical activity; positive and negative affects	Palm Pilot Zire 22	7 days	8	Randomized	75%	No	Both samples show higher PA following physical activity. More specifically, depressed patients show a significantly higher increase in experienced PA levels after physical activity.
	[32]	MDD (n = 14) and HCG (n = 43)	Mood; physical symptoms; phyoical activity	Ruputer ECOLOG	Average: 37.43 days (range:18–67 days)	4	Semi-randomized	93%	Ambulatory Monitors Inc.—actigraph	Depressive mood is associated with increased intermittency of locomotor activity.
	[37]	MDD (n = 10), and HCG (n = 10)	Mood; cognition; daily activities; physical activity	PsyMate	30 days	3	Fixed sampling scheme	91%	ActiCal Respironics—actigraph	Despite the observation of large interindividual differences, results show a positive effect of physical activity on PA in all participants.
Rumination	[51]	MDD (n = 6) and HCG (n = 7)	Context; mood; depressive symptoms; EEG (at baseline)	Palm Pilot and EEG (at baseline)	7 days	5	Not specified	Not specified	No	Lower activation of bilateral PFC predicts higher rates of rumination, whereas higher levels of self-esteem are associated with lower right PFC activity.
	[35]	MDD (n = 18) and HCG (n = 18)	Thoughts; disturbing events; feelings; possible influencing factors; feelings; HR	Electronic diary implemented on a smartphone	1 day	Not reported	Semi-randomized	Not specified	RS 800CX; Bodyguard2 (HR and HRV)	Depressed participants show higher rates of perseverative cognition, which are associated with lower HRV.
	[52]	MDD (n = 38), GAD (n = 36), MDD with GAD comorbidity (n = 38), and HCG (n = 33)	Events stressfulness; rumination	Palm Pilot Zire 22	7 days	8	Randomized	72%	No	MDD and GAD participants show the same level of rumination, which is even more severe in comorbid cases. Higher rates of rumination are predictive of worse affect, more maladaptive behaviours, and more severe symptoms.
	[53]	MDD (n = 16), GAD (n = 15), MDD with GAD comorbidity (n = 20), and HCG (n = 19)	Rumination; worry; PA and NA; significant events	Palm Pilot Zire 22	6 to7 days	8	Semi-randomized	65%	No	Levels of rumination among all the clinical samples are higher in response to significant events. Decreased PA and increased NA are associated with higher momentary rumination.

Table 2. *Cont.*

	Authors	Sample	Variables	Device(s)	Duration	Prompts Per Day	Sampling Schema	Compliance	Sensor(s)	Primary Outcome(s)
Emotional reaction	[54]	Remitted MDD (n = 55) and HCG (n = 55)	Perceived stress; mood	Hand held Psion "Revo" computer	7 days	5	Randomized	90%	No	Past episodes of depression are likely to increase the vulnerability to stressful events, especially in male participants.
	[55]	MDD (n = 35), mD (n = 26), and HCG (n = 38)	Context; mood; events (nature of the event; location; people involved; affective rating)	Palm Pilot Zire 22	3 non-consecutive days (over a period of 5 days)	10	Semi-randomized	65%	No	Both MDD and mD patients show lower levels of positive affect and rate events as more stressful and unpleasant than the control group. Furthermore, they show a higher reduction in negative feelings after positive events.
	[50]	MDD (n = 53), and HCG (n = 53)	Affect; significant events	Palm Pilot Zire 22	7/8 days	8	Randomized	78%	No	Results point out greater emotional instability with respect to NA in depressed patients. No differences are observed in terms of reactivity, inertia, and instability in PA.
	[56]	MDD (n = 21) and MDD with BPD comorbidity (n = 20)	Affect and mood; events; subjective affective reactivity	Smartphone to access a web platform	7 days	5	Randomized	94%	No	Comorbidity with BPD does not imply major affective instability, but it is associated with lower subjective perception of affective reactivity.
	[57]	Remitted MDD (n = 10) and HCG (n = 11)	Mood; PA and NA; visual mental imagery	"Imagine your Mood", smartphone application	3 days a week, for 8 weeks	10	Semi-randomized	Not specified	No	In both samples, higher levels of visual imagery-based processing are associated with higher levels of PA and better mood, regardless of the valence of the imagery content. Elevated levels of visual imagery-based processing are not associated with daily affective reactivity.
	[58]	MDD (n = 51), and BPD (n = 80)	PA, NA, fear; hostility; sadness; interpersonal events	Palm Pilot Zire 31	28 days	6	Semi-randomized	86%	No	Rejection and disagreement increase NA (especially hostility and sadness) both at a momentary and daily level, regardless of the diagnosis. The association between rejection/disagreement and hostility is stronger in BPD patients.
	[59]	MDD (n = 12), DD (n = 3), BD (n = 15)	Affect; location; social context; gambling desire/motivation/activities	Palm Pilot Zire 22	30 days	3	Randomized	73%	No	High levels of sadness and arousal are predictive of gambling desire, regardless of the diagnosis. Depressed individuals are likely to gamble to increase PA or for social reasons.
	[60]	MDD (n = 15), GAD (n = 25)	Symptoms, PA, NA, rumination, behavioural avoidance, reassurance seeking	Web-based survey	30 days	4	Not specified	Not specified	No	Using a person by person approach, results show that moment-to-moment symptomatology is mainly driven by positive mood, hopelessness, anger, and irritability, but not depressed mood, anhedonia, or worry.

MDD: major depressive disorder; mD: minor depression; HCG: healthy control group; BDP: borderline personality disorder; GAD: generalized anxiety disorders; PDA: personal digital assistant; DD: dysthymic disorder; PFC: prefrontal cortex; PA: positive affect; NA: negative affect; HRV: heart rate variability; PHQ-9: Patient Health Questionnaire-9; QUID-SR: Quick Inventory of Depressive Symptomatology—Self Report; HADS-A: Hospital Anxiety and Depression Scale; PANAS: Positive and Negative Affect Schedule; HPAA: hypothalamic-pituitary-adrenal axis.

Table 3. More detailed information about the selected Ecological Momentary Intervention studies.

Authors	Name	Sample	Intervention	Duration	Prompts	Sampling Schema	Sensor(s)	Primary Outcome(s)
[61]	Mobylize!	MDD (n = 7), with different comorbidities	Mobylize! is a context-aware system, composed of three main elements: (1) A mobile application for the collection of self-reports; (2) a website with feedback and theoretical lessons; (3) periodic contacts with trained coaches	8 weeks	5/day	Randomized	38 concurrent sensors integrated in the phone	Mobylize! significantly reduced depressive symptoms. Predictive models did not reach high levels of accuracy, especially for mood.
[62]	PsyMate	MDD (n = 102): Experimental condition (n = 33), pseudo-experimental condition (n = 36), control condition (n = 33)	Daily assessment of self-reports and weekly EMA-derived feedback through face-to-face sessions	3 days per week, for 6 weeks	10/day	Semi-randomized	No	The use of EMA-derived feedback as a complementary intervention to pharmacological treatment significantly decreased depressive symptoms. These improvements were also maintained over time.
[63]	PsyMate	MDD (n = 102): Experimental condition (n = 33), pseudo-experimental condition (n = 36), control condition (n = 33)	Daily assessment of self-reports and weekly EMA-derived feedback through face-to-face sessions	3 days per week, for 6 weeks	10/day	Semi-randomized	No	The use of Psymate as a technique of self-monitoring could improve patients' feelings of empowerment.
[64]	PsyMate	MDD (n = 102): Experimental condition (n = 33), pseudo-experimental condition (n = 36), control condition (n = 33)	Daily assessment of self-reports and weekly EMA-derived feedback through face-to-face sessions	3 days per week, for 6 weeks	10/day	Semi-randomized	No	Face-to-face EMA-derived feedback sessions did not increase the rate of PA experienced during or shortly after the intervention.
[65]	Medlink	MDD (n = 8)	Medlink is a mobile application delivering psychological support to MDD patients. The application provides users with: (1) psychoeducation; (2) weekly symptom assessment; (3) medication adherence monitoring; (4) monthly communication with a professional based on the previous points	4 weeks	1/week	Not specified	No	Medlink was positively evaluated by participants, especially regarding the weekly psychoeducation lessons. Depression severity of participants significantly decreased over the course of the experiment.

Table 3. *Cont.*

Author	Name	Sample	Intervention	Duration	Prompts	Sampling Schema	Sensor(s)	Primary Outcome(s)
[66]	Help4Mood	MDD (n = 28): Experimental condition (n = 14) and control condition (n = 14)	Web platform providing daily assessment of symptoms, self-monitoring, and tailored activities. The delivered content is created in response to the user's actions through a virtual agent	About 5 weeks	CESD-VAS-VA: 1/day PHQ-9: 1/week	Not specified	Accelerometer and acoustic speech analysis	Only half of the participants used Help4Mood regularly. Significant changes in depressive symptoms were observed only among regular users.
[67]	PsyMate	MDD (n = 102): Experimental condition (n = 33), pseudo-experimental condition (n = 36), control condition (n = 33)	Daily assessment of self-reports and weekly EMA-derived feedback through face-to-face sessions	3 days per week, for 6 weeks	10/day	Semi-randomized	No	The use of EMA-derived feedback decreased depressive symptoms and improved maladaptive behaviours.
[68]	PsyMate	MDD (n = 79): Experimental condition (n = 25), pseudo-experimental condition (n = 30), control condition (n = 24)	Daily assessment of self-reports and weekly EMA-derived feedback through face-to-face sessions	3 days per week, for 6 weeks	10/day	Semi-randomized	No	The use of a self-monitoring EMA improves negative emotion differentiation.

MDD: major depressive disorder; PA: positive affect; CESD-VAS-VA: brief visual analogue scale version of the Center of Epidemiological Studies Depression. Scale; PHQ-9: Patient Health Questionnaire.

3.1.2. Sampling Methods

Currently, different EMA designs can be used to define prompt scheduling, depending on the main purpose of the study. It is possible to prompt participants using fixed time periods or randomized/semi-randomized samplings (time-based sampling). Alternatively, participants can be asked to personally fill in the assessment after the occurrence of a specific behaviour or event (event-based sampling). Whereas time-based samplings depend on a signal emitted by the device (signal-contingent), event-based samplings are not preceded by a prompt (event-contingent). Signal-contingent schemas are useful when repeated measures are needed to obtain a representative value of a variable or when the objective is to capture dynamic variables (e.g., mood), whereas event-contingent schemas are more likely to be adopted when the main focus is on a specific behaviour that occurs randomly or less frequently during the day (e.g., smoking a cigarette). Regarding our selected studies, none of them adopted event-based sampling. Most of the studies collected data using randomized or semi-randomized schemas, whereas nine studies prompted participants to note information at fixed time points during the day. This latter approach was adopted especially by the studies that investigated the association between cortisol or melatonin and depression, i.e., when the assessed variable required greater temporal precision and accuracy.

The duration of the data collection showed great variability. Some studies collected self-reports for a brief time period (less than 3 days); this choice was especially observed in the field of cortisol and sleep pattern research. Other studies required longer periods of assessment, where participants were involved for one or two months. This was especially true for studies investigating physical activity and its association with depressive symptoms. The same high variability was observed in the number of prompts, which varied from 1 to 20 prompts per day.

3.1.3. Compliance and Dropout Rates

With the term "compliance", we refer to the percentage of answered prompts. A few studies did not report this information [35,40–42,51,57,60]. However, the majority clearly addressed this issue. Sixteen studies reported compliance rates higher than 85%, five studies showed rates between 84% and 70%, and four studies collected 65% of the total possible answers. Patient dropout was related to diagnosis change, subjective burden, technical problems, incomplete data, retrospective completion of the electronic diary, missed prompts, worsening of symptoms, or non-attendance at follow-up sessions.

To prevent backfilling, different solutions were adopted. In most of the studies, participants could complete self-reports for a fixed time period after the prompt, ranging from a few minutes to a maximum of one hour. To increase compliance, two studies also gave participants the possibility of postponing prompts.

3.1.4. Contribution of EMA to the Study of MDD

As Table 4 shows, so far EMA has been applied to seven different fields. In the following paragraph, we will provide an overview of EMA's contribution to the understanding and assessment of MDD.

Table 4. Fields of application of EMAs for Major Depressive Disorder.

Field of Application	Retrieved Articles	Aim	Advantages
Recall bias	[8,26]	Experimental	No retrospective bias; control over backfilling; repeated momentary measurements.
Symptoms monitoring	[39–41]	Clinical	Continuous monitoring (symptoms assessment, treatment progress); real-time feedback to clinicians (e.g., crisis plan) and users (e.g., patterns visualization).

Table 4. *Cont.*

Field of Application	Retrieved Articles	Aim	Advantages
Cortisol dysregulation	[31,36,42–45]	Experimental	Role of contextual variables; temporal relationship between physiological measures and self-reports.
Sleep patterns	[33,38,46–49]	Experimental	Control over backfilling; no retrospective bias; integration of self-reports with passive data supplied by sensors and biosensors.
Physical activity	[32,37,50]	Experimental	Role of contextual variables; integration of self-reports with passive data supplied by sensors; temporal relationship between physiological measures and self-reports.
Rumination	[35,51–53]	Experimental	Role of contextual variables; rumination deployment across time.
Affect and emotional reactivity	[50,54–60],	Experimental	Role of contextual variables; temporal deployment of affect and emotional reactivity.

Recall Bias

Increasing evidence shows that memories often have inaccurate and imprecise content due to recall bias. In the case of EMAs, two studies were carried out to investigate this bias, comparing EMA daily data to retrospective assessments. Ben-Zeev and colleagues compared positive (PA) and negative (NA) affect collected through an EMA to scores obtained by means of traditional paper-and-pencil retrospective questionnaires [8]. When retrospectively recalled, both PA and NA were overestimated, regardless of the diagnosis. Interestingly, the control group was more likely to exaggerate the retrieval of PA rather than NA, but this trend was not observed in depressed patients. By contrast, Torous and colleagues developed a smartphone application to administer randomized subsets of items taken from the Patient Health Questionnaire (PHQ-9) [69], compared to the traditional paper-based PHQ-9. Symptoms were evaluated as more severe in daily EMA evaluations, compared to the retrospective PHQ-9 assessment. According to the authors, this discrepancy could be due to different factors, such as recall bias or stigma.

Symptom Monitoring

Unexpectedly, we could only retrieve three studies within this research field, i.e., studies that actually applied EMA to monitor clinically depressed patients. Husky and colleagues investigated the acceptability of a three-days computerized ambulatory monitoring on MDD and BD patients, showing encouraging compliance and acceptance rates among both samples. Practice effects were observed (faster response time over the course of the study), thus suggesting the importance of considering the potential effects of EMA duration on self-reports [39]. Schaffer et al. developed a system called "Mental Health Telemetry" to monitor symptoms of patients receiving pharmacological treatment [40]. According to the results, a reduction in depressive symptoms was already observable one day after beginning the treatment, and symptoms on day 7 were predictive of treatment outcome. Similarly, iHOPE is a smartphone application for the daily monitoring of depressive symptoms and sleep patterns [41]. EMA assessments of depression, sleep quality, and anxiety were highly associated with the Hamilton Depression Rating Scale (HAM-D), administered at baseline. Nevertheless, application use decreased significantly over the weeks, from 3.4 days per week to 0.4 days per week after 8 weeks, highlighting the important issue of compliance in EMA assessments.

Cortisol Secretion

Stetler and colleagues investigated the associations among cortisol and sleep patterns, social interactions [43], and daily activities [42]. Not only were cortisol levels after awakening different in depressed and healthy participants, but the impact of psychosocial variables on cortisol secretion was also dissimilar. Consistently, the Hypothalamic–pituitary–adrenal (HPA) axis of depressed patients was no longer able to respond to the timing of the sleep-wake cycle, daily routines, and external social experiences. One study explored the impact of cortisol on affect, showing a bidirectional association between PA and NA and daily cortisol levels [45]. Nevertheless, high variability was observed among participants regarding the timing, direction, and sign of this association. For instance, NA was positively associated with cortisol 50% of the time, while the association between cortisol and PA was almost always negative. Booij et al. identified higher cortisol and α-amylase levels among depressed individuals [36]. Similarly, when applying individual correction for lifestyle factors, the association of depression to cortisol and the ratio of α-amylase over cortisol was no longer significant, suggesting that generalization from groups does not always reflect the single individual. Nevertheless, Conrad and colleagues could not find cortisol differences between depressed and non-depressed participants. Interestingly, a negative correlation between NA and heart rate variability (HRV) was observed only in the control group, suggesting that constant NA may alter the normal interaction between affectivity and the autonomic nervous system [31].

Finally, interesting outcomes were also observed among remitted MDD patients [44]. Despite remission, patients showed reduced cortisol levels throughout the day and a different interaction between affect and cortisol, thus suggesting a reduction in the HPA axis' responsiveness as a potential marker of recurrent depression.

Sleep Patterns

According to our search, six studies adopted an EMA to explore sleep disturbances in depression. Through the daily administration of morning self-reports about sleep patterns, O'Leary et al. found that depression was associated with lower perceived sleep quality, which in turn affected negative emotional reactivity to both neutral and unpleasant events during the day [47]. However, in healthy participants, sleep disturbances only affected emotional reactivity to unpleasant events. In other words, depression could be a factor affecting the relationship between sleep quality and emotional reactivity. Similarly, two studies analysed the influence of sleep quality on daily affect [46,48]. As expected, higher sleep quality was associated with higher PA in both healthy and depressed participants. Surprisingly, there was no evidence of the moderating role of depression in the association between sleep and affect. Nevertheless, sleep quality affected daily mood, but not vice versa, because higher sleep quality was associated with increased PA and decreased NA the following day. This association did not differ between depressed and healthy participants. Similarly, sleep duration was found to affect next-day physical activity, but again, no difference between depressed and non-depressed individuals was observed [38]. An EMA was finally adopted to investigate the association between sleep patterns and suicide ideation in a sample of depressed patients [33]. Poor sleep quality, both at subjective and objective levels, was associated with increased suicide ideations the following day. However, suicidal thoughts did not predict sleep patterns the following night.

Bouwmans and colleagues also collected repeated saliva samples to analyse the association of depression with melatonin, an important hormone related to sleep onset [49]. A bidirectional relationship between affect and fatigue, and melatonin was pointed out: Melatonin is associated with changes in affect and fatigue; however, affect and fatigue are also predictors of melatonin levels. Participants that did not show this association were likely to report higher rates of depression, worse sleep quality, and lower energy expenditure.

Physical Activity

In order to analyse the effect of self-initiated physical activity on mood, clinically depressed patients were asked to report their daily physical activity [50]. Both healthy and depressed participants showed higher levels of PA following physical activity, but no decrease in NA. Notably, the increase in PA after physical exercise was greater in depressed patients, which is consistent with the ample evidence supporting behavioural activation in general, and physical activity in particular, for the treatment of depression. Confirming these results, another study found that physical activity was associated with subsequent increased PA, regardless of the diagnosis [37]. However, the analysis also revealed high subjective variability in the association between physical activity and mood in terms of strength, direction, and temporal aspects. Finally, Kim and colleagues developed a statistical model with cross validity that identified a significant association between higher intermittency of locomotor activity and worse mood ratings [32], suggesting the possibility of predicting patients' moods through the analysis of momentary locomotor patterns. According to their model, a worsening of depressive mood was associated with increased intermittency of locomotor activity.

Rumination

Ruscio and colleagues investigated the relationship between stressful events and rumination in MDD and GAD patients [52]. Both clinical samples showed higher levels of rumination in response to stressful situations, which were further worsened by symptom severity and extensive comorbidity. In addition, rumination significantly mediated the impact of stress on symptoms and affect; that is, higher rumination after a stressful event predicted greater NA and more maladaptive behaviours. Putman and colleagues investigated rumination and self-esteem through the assessment of resting baseline PFC alpha activity, along with the momentary assessment of affect and depressive symptoms, in a sample of clinically depressed individuals [51]. Rumination was found to be associated with an increased alpha signal in the bilateral prefrontal cortex (i.e., decreased neural activation), whereas an increased alpha signal in the right prefrontal cortex was positively correlated with higher self-esteem ratings. One study investigated perseverative thoughts (i.e., depressive rumination, worry, and reactive rumination) in relation to mind wandering [35]. Participants were instructed to complete a smartphone diary every 30 min for one day, and these self-reports were integrated with continuous HR monitoring. Confirming the hypothesis that mind wandering is not a maladaptive behaviour per se, only perseverative cognition was associated with health risk factors, such as lower HRV, worse mood, and higher interference in daily functioning. Finally, one study examined the dynamics of worry and rumination in daily life [53]. Contrary to the hypothesis, levels of worry were not significantly associated with the occurrence of significant events, whereas rumination was significantly higher in response to these circumstances. Compared to the control group, clinically depressed individuals showed decreased PA and increased NA as a consequence of high rumination levels.

Affect and Emotional Reactivity

Thompson and colleagues investigated emotional reactivity, emotional inertia, and emotional instability in depressed patients [50]. Compared to healthy participants, clinically depressed patients showed higher NA instability, whereas no differences in PA instability were observed. Both samples reported increased NA after a negative event; however, depressed patients showed a greater decrease in NA and increase in PA after a positive event. These results were confirmed by another study that showed a greater reduction in NA following positive events in depressed individuals [55]. When considering BPD comorbidity, depressed patients were found to be less emotionally influenced by events, and to perceive themselves as less emotionally reactive [56]. Other factors that affect emotional reactivity are gender and past depression [54]. In one study, women and remitted patients evaluated daily events as more negative than men, and they showed worse mood and higher emotional reactivity in response to daily stressors. Finally, a smartphone application was developed to assess visual mental imagery and its impact on mood and affective reactivity in healthy people and remitted MDD patients [57]. Participants were asked to focus on their mental representations, i.e., what they had in mind, eight times per day. Imagery-based processing was associated with better mood, regardless of the valence of the mental representation. This pattern was similar in healthy and depressed participants. However, no association between mental imagery and affective reactivity was observed.

Regarding daily affect, one study explored the impact of gambling desire on mood in a sample of depressed individuals [59]. Higher levels of sadness and arousal were associated with higher rates of gambling desire. Consistently, depressed participants were also likely to perform gambling behaviours to increase their current PA levels. However, momentary affect did not predict actual gambling behaviours. An EMA was also used to investigate the influence of social rejection and disagreement on daily affect in MDD and BPD patients [58]. As expected, momentary and daily negative interpersonal events triggered higher NA (fear, hostility, and sadness) in both groups. High levels of hostility predicted rejection and disagreements, whereas sadness was only a predictor of social rejection. The aforementioned relationships were stronger in BPD patients than in depressed participants.

Finally, one study investigated the topology and temporal dynamics of depression and anxiety symptoms using contemporaneous and temporal network models [60]. Positive (positive, content, enthusiastic, energetic) and negative (down) mood were the most representative variables of patients' core symptoms. While "worried" and "down" did not show temporal influence, "positive mood", "hopelessness", "anger", and "irritability" were the strongest drivers of moment-to-moment symptomatology.

3.2. *Ecological Momentary Intervention in MDD*

The selection process resulted in eight studies that administered an EMI to clinically depressed patients. In all, four different interventions were identified: Psymate, Mobylize, Hel4Mood, and Medlink.

3.2.1. General Overview of the Interventions

Psymate is a PDA-based EMA for symptom monitoring that aims to increase awareness about depression and the dynamics that characterize this disorder [62–64,67,68]. Psymate allows patients to record daily symptoms and affect. Based on these daily assessments, patients meet a clinician weekly and receive graphical feedback on the association between PA levels and daily life activities, events, or social interactions, as well as on the association between PA changes and the number of depressive complaints. In this way, patients have the chance to reflect on their affective state and the relationship between symptoms and contextual variables with a professional. According to Heron's definition, "the key feature of all EMIs is that the treatment is provided to people during their everyday lives (i.e., in real time) and settings (i.e., real world)" [22]. Therefore, Psymate does not meet all the criteria for an EMI, as EMA-feedbacks are provided during weekly face-to-face sessions. However, we decided to include this intervention because we think it provides important insights about the potential of self-monitoring EMA as a therapeutic tool.

Likewise, Mobylize! constitutes an ecological intervention composed of a mobile application, an interactive website, and a system for email/telephone support [61]. The most innovative aspect of this application is the integration of self-reports with data from smartphone sensors. Mobylize! is provided with a context-aware system. Thanks to a machine learning algorithm, the application can predict the state of the patient (mood, emotions, cognitive/motivational states, activities, environmental context, and social context). Specifically, the system works in three different phases: (1) Data collection, during which 38 sensors collect sensor information; (2) learners, during which prompted self-reports are matched and paired with simultaneously labelled state data to develop predictive models; and (3) action components, a continuous process that analyses sensor data in order to update previous predictive models without the direct input of the user. Mobylize! is designed to prompt patients to assess mood, intensity of emotions, fatigue, pleasure, accomplishment, concentration, engagement, perceived control, location, and interactions five or more times a day. To accommodate new data, every new self-report is subsequently associated with the generation and modification of previous models. Thanks to this complex system, the mobile application sends tailored feedback to participants. Through the website, users can graphically visualize self-report patterns, read theoretical lessons, and use interactive tools, such as tailored plans and calendars, for monitoring daily activities. Lastly, a trained clinician contacts users periodically by phone or email to provide technical support, reinforce adherence, and enhance motivation.

Help4Mood is a web-platform to self-monitor daily symptoms, mood, activities, and thoughts [66]. Based on a Cognitive Behavioural Therapy (CBT) approach, Help4Mood helps patients to reflect on the emotional and cognitive patterns related to depression. In addition to collecting daily self-reports, the application receives data from an actimetry sensor and acoustic analysis of speech. The innovative aspect of Help4Mood is the use of a virtual agent, completely customizable in terms of voice, clothing style, sex, and language, that communicates with users to provide tailored exercises and activities and guide them through the daily questionnaires. The application also has an emergency section called the "crisis plan": As soon as symptom worsening is detected, the application prompts users to contact a professional or a relative.

Finally, Medlink is a mobile application to support and monitor MDD patients taking antidepressant medication [65]. The main purpose of the app is to address the failure points that usually occur between professionals and newly diagnosed patients. On the one hand, the application provides users with weekly psychoeducation material and sends suggestions about medication management and how to deal with depressive symptoms. On the other hand, it monitors patients' treatment and depressive symptoms. Every four weeks, personal communication with a professional is scheduled to give patients monthly feedback about disease progression.

3.2.2. Effectiveness of the Intervention

Psymate was tested in a sample of 102 clinically depressed patients in a three-arm randomized controlled trial [62–64,67] with an experimental condition (treatment as usual – TAU - and six-week Psymate treatment, with weekly face-to-face feedback sessions), a pseudo-experimental condition (TAU and Psymate without EMA face-to-face feedbacks), and a control condition (TAU). Three different categories of weekly feedback were provided: (1) Positive affect, (2) positive affect in relation to events appraised with an internal versus external locus of control, and (3) positive affect in relation to social interactions. Results showed a significant reduction in depressive symptoms in the experimental group that was maintained in the follow-up assessment. Participants in the pseudo-experimental condition reported decreased depressive symptoms in the first weeks of the treatment, but this gain was not maintained across the weeks. Notably, the use of Psymate was associated with increased levels of perceived empowerment, regardless of the presence of weekly feedback, and with increased experienced PA throughout the treatment. Decreased depressive symptoms were also associated with increased positive daily behaviours. Finally, Widdershoven and colleagues observed a significant improvement in negative emotions' differentiation and a close-to-significance improvement in positive emotions' differentiation after 6-weeks of self-monitoring, regardless of EMA-derived feedbacks [68].

Mobylize! was tested in a small pilot study with a sample of 7 MMD patients [61]. According to the results, the use of Mobylize! significantly reduced depressive symptoms, both on a self-rated measure (PHQ-9) and a clinician-based evaluation (Quick Inventory of Depressive Symptomatology-Clinician Rating, QUIDS-C), as well as anxiety symptoms, measured with the Generalized Anxiety Disorder Scale (GAD-7). At the end of the treatment, participants were also less likely to meet MDD diagnostic criteria. Nevertheless, the accuracy of the predictive model was low, especially for mood; higher accuracy was achieved by models that predicted location, conversational state, and social interactions (accuracy between 60% and 90%).

A randomized controlled trial was conducted to evaluate Help4Mood [66]. Twenty-eight depressed patients were recruited and randomized into two treatment groups: Help4Mood and TAU. Outcome measures, which included the Beck Depression Inventory (BDI) and Quick Inventory of Depressive Symptomatology—Self Report (QIDS-SR), indicated reduced symptoms in both samples. Nevertheless, patients in the TAU group achieved greater clinical improvement compared to patients who used the application. Notably, regular users were more likely to obtain greater clinical improvement compared to users with low compliance.

Finally, a preliminary study tested the efficacy of Medlink with 8 MDD patients [65]. On the one hand, medication monitoring showed promising outcomes. Patients reported taking 84% of their medication, which is significantly higher than medication adherence rates reported in the literature. On the other hand, depressive symptoms significantly decreased over the course of 4 weeks.

3.2.3. Compliance and Dropout Rates

Regarding Psymate, the number of answered prompts in both the experimental and pseudo-experimental groups was 135.5 out of 180 (75.3%); participants completed 39.7 out of 50 pre-assessments (79.4%) and 23.7 out of 30 (79%) post-assessment observations. Moreover, 27 of the 33 participants (81.9%) allocated to the experimental group completed the intervention, whereas 32 out of 36 participants (88.89%) allocated to the pseudo-experimental group completed it.

Throughout the 8-week treatment with Mobylize, the mean number of log-ins to the mobile application was 7.9 (approximately one per week), whereas the number of completed lessons on the website was 4.8 out of 9 (53.3%). The number of answered prompts drastically decreased throughout the treatment, from 15.3 in the first week to 4.8 in the last week, due to technical difficulties and connectivity problems. Seven out of eight participants (87.5%) completed the intervention: The only dropout was caused by technical problems with the smartphone.

Regarding Help4Mood, the authors indicated great variability in terms of time of use. Two participants used the application for one or two days, whereas three participants used it between 3 and 7 days. The remaining six participants used it more than 10 times, approximately twice a week. The mean use was 134 min. Eleven out of 13 (84.6%) participants completed the protocol and were assessed for the follow-up. One participant withdrew due to worsening mood.

Finally, participants entered the Medlink application approximately 17.4 times during the 4 weeks of data collection and answered 96% of the prompts. Seven out of nine users read the psychoeducation lessons from the first and second week, whereas only half of them read the third and fourth lessons. No dropouts were reported.

3.2.4. Participants' Feedback and Satisfaction

Using Likert scales ranging from 1 to 7, participants found that Psymate was very simple to use and provided clear instructions (verbal instructions = 6.6 ± 0.7; written instructions = 6.5 ± 1.0; Psymate answers = 2.6 ± 1.5). The number of daily prompts and the time needed to complete assessments was not stressful (number of beeps per day = 3.1 ± 1.6; time to answer = 2.5 ± 1.5). Finally, satisfaction with its most important feature, i.e., receiving EMA-derived feedback, indicated that the feedback was highly appreciated (usefulness of feedback = 6.2 ± 0.7) and considered valuable (feedback to improve daily skills = 5.4 ± 1.1). However, participants would have appreciated receiving more specific and practical advice related to the EMA-based feedback (3.2 ± 2.0).

Regarding Mobylize, satisfaction with the application was rated as 5.71 on a scale from 1 to 7. Criticism was related to technical problems, such as loss of connectivity and subsequent failure to receive prompts. Interestingly, 86% of the participants reported that the intervention was particularly helpful for identifying NA triggers and avoiding distressing and maladaptive behaviours. Participants also suggested lengthening the intervention and adding more activities, such as a blog to talk with other users or a message service between patients and coaches.

Participants involved in the Help4Mood study were quite satisfied with the application. Most of them would use it in everyday life and suggest it to other patients. The idea of a virtual agent to guide participants in completing the assessments was appreciated; however, some participants perceived the agent as too cold, repetitive, and not sufficiently realistic. Among the limitations, patients reported sometimes being bored by excessively long sessions. They would have appreciated receiving more psychoeducational material and a more tailored experience, allowing them to access their preferred materials and activities without restrictions.

Medlink's usability was assessed using 4 items from the Usefulness, Satisfaction, and Ease of Use Questionnaire (USE). On a scale from 1 to 7, participants reported encouraging scores for ease of use (mean = 5.7 ± 1.1) and learnability (mean = 6.1 ± 1.5), but low scores for perceived usefulness (mean = 4.6 ± 1.0) and satisfaction (mean = 4.8 ± 0.8). Furthermore, encouraging ratings were observed for the weekly psychoeducation lessons (liking = 6.0 ± 1.1; ease of use = 6.6 ± 0.5; learnability = 6.6 ± 0.5; and usefulness = 5.8 ± 1.7), which were also reported to be the most interesting and useful parts of the application. Finally, feedback interviews showed neutral comments regarding daily self-reports, that were perceived as not very useful; contrasting opinions were collected regarding feedback graphs.

4. Discussion

To date, the scientific literature has mostly been based on studies conducted in laboratory settings, thus understudying the daily dynamics of psychopathology [70]. Therefore, unobtrusively monitoring behavioural (i.e., sensors), physiological (i.e., biosensors), and cognitive/emotional (i.e., self-reports) factors in ecological settings collected through portable and wearable devices can provide new information about elusive psychological constructs that are usually defined by the complex dynamics of contexts and variability. Accordingly, the research field could benefit from the use of novel technologies to better explore MDD mechanisms and delineate new theoretical models based on ecological observations.

Compared to paper and pencil daily diaries, the use of electronic devices, and especially smartphones, could further increase the six EMA advantages identified by Ebner-Premier (Table 5) [16]: (a) The automation of the entire process directly on a mobile device, such as a smartphone, can provide greater control over backfilling and higher temporal precision in the administration, planning, and randomization of prompts; (b) the use of ICTs can offer additional possibilities for multimodal assessments, with data supplied by embedded sensors and wearable unobstructed biosensors that can automatically be coordinated with the collection of self-reports; (c) the use of mobile devices reduces the effort required of users in completing daily assessments and prevents errors by researchers and clinicians due to manual data entry; (d) smartphones offer the possibility of providing real-time EMA-derived feedback that can be an important therapeutic tool for patients' self-monitoring, in addition to the possibility of sending real-time alerts to clinicians in case of need. In this regard, smartphones have the potential of becoming global low-cost tools that can also be adopted in the clinical field. Currently, 2.32 billion people in the world use smartphones, and it has been estimated that, by 2020, 70% of the world's population will own one [71]. The potential of these devices is also supported by the evidence showing that people with serious mental and physical illnesses own and regularly use smartphones [72] and are interested in using applications for their health [26].

As pointed out in this review, the widespread adoption of EMA for the investigation of depression has led to novel insights into different aspects of the disease, including emotion reactivity, cortisol patterns, or daily rumination. We discussed different sampling methods that can be used in EMA protocols, showing that the signal-contingent design with prompt randomization or semi-randomization is the most widely adopted option when dealing with variables, such as affect and symptom monitoring. We also reported compliance and dropout rates, which showed encouraging results, with most of the studies reporting more than 70% adherence. Nevertheless, the gap between clinical practice and research is still quite wide, as revealed by the low number of studies that adopt this approach to assess and monitor patients for clinical purposes or implement EMA in clinical settings. Accordingly, many issues still need to be addressed. To date, no standard and validated sets of items have been developed for EMA protocols, raising the problem of context validity. Moreover, further research should be conducted to improve patients' compliance and reduce dropout. Due to the intrinsic nature of the disease, depressed patients could be less likely to consistently complete daily assessments. In a previous study, we observed that compliance was higher in EMA administered through a smartphone and when patients were prompted less than 8 times a day [73]. However, a meta-analysis should be conducted to more precisely identify the factors that improve adherence (see, for example, [74]), thus providing some sort of guideline for the design of EMA. Indeed, we strongly believe that clinical practice could benefit from the use of EMAs for several reasons. First, EMAs can be useful for diagnostic purposes. Traditional diagnostic procedures usually involve a static moment in time, including semi-structured interviews (e.g., Mini-International Neuropsychiatric Interview) complemented by self-report measures. However, ample evidence shows the dynamic nature of affective states and mood [75]. Furthermore, these dynamics greatly vary from person to person, reasons for which ideographic approaches may shed light upon the structure of individual symptom dynamics [60]. Consequently, by means of EMAs, a more accurate diagnostic process could be pursued. Likewise, the continuous monitoring of patients' symptoms would allow clinicians to monitor the efficacy of a treatment over time [76], predict short-term mood changes [77], detect symptoms' worsening in an early stage [78], and create continuous communication between clinicians and patients. On the other hand, the use of daily mood and symptom self-ratings could provide more ecological assessments, overcoming recall bias and capturing the dynamics of human functioning in daily life that cannot be detected with traditional tools.

Table 5. Benefits of using EMA for mood dysregulation and mood disorders as described by Ebner-Premier [16].

	Advantages	Implications
1	Real-time assessments	Reduction in retrospective bias and increase in accuracy.
2	Repeated measurements	Better comprehension of time-dependent processes and dynamic changes in symptoms.
3	Multimodal assessments	Contemporary analysis of behaviours, physiological signals, and subjective experiences.
4	Context-specific information	Assessment of symptoms as context-dependent.
5	Interactive assessments	Real-time customizable and interactive feedback.
6	Generalizability	Higher ecological validity and collection of more representative data.

Our results also highlight the existence of a small number of EMIs for depression. In the current literature, only four ecological interventions have been developed, and only two of them were tested in a randomized-controlled trial (RCT). Our review showed promising results in terms of patient satisfaction and clinical efficacy, further supporting the need for more efforts in this direction. However, compliance rates were sometimes not encouraging, and a major challenge is to encourage regular use of these technologies throughout the entire treatment process [79]. Accordingly, future research should focus on the concept of users' motivation and engagement, taking into consideration the adoption of focus groups with patients during treatments, using mixed quantitative and qualitative designs to obtain as much information as possible to guide future developments, and extending the effects of gamification features on adherence and compliance [80]. In other words, greater attention should be paid to the needs and characteristics of the target population. Considering feedback from users, here, we were able to identify three EMI features that were highly appreciated: The possibility of receiving visual feedback about daily assessments and, therefore, self-monitoring of daily patterns;

the availability of psychoeducational material on depression and its mechanisms; and the opportunity to have continuous or periodic communication with a trained clinician.

In this review, we found that most of the EMAs were based only on self-reports, whereas more attempts to integrate this information with data gathered from sensors and biosensors were observed for EMIs. Recent advances in sensor technologies have had an impact on applications for remote health [81], such as postoperative recovery [82], treatment for chronic patients [83], and monitoring of elderly individuals [84]. Consistently, the hierarchical sensing model proposed by Mohr highlights the great revolution that new sensors and biosensors can bring to the field of mental health [85], making it possible to collect raw sensor data (i.e., the lower level of the hierarchy) that can be converted into "behavioural markers" through machine learning and data mining methods [18].

Smartphone sensors further increase the potentially collectable information, allowing the reconstruction of people's habits, sleep patterns, or social life by using embedded sensors, such as accelerometers, calls, short message service (SMS), social network data, or geolocation. In other words, it is now possible to infer and collect behavioural information without necessarily asking the person to report it.

Even though they were not investigated in the studies targeted at MDD patients discussed here, several opportunities can be found in the integration of EMA and EMI platforms with behavioural and physiological signal processing, further mediated by machine learning algorithms. On the one hand, several behavioural signals are readily collectable with the use of smartphone sensors, even though they may lack the required specificity for mood recognition and prediction, as found by the Mobylize! study [61]. On the other hand, due to recent advancements in sensor technologies, physiological signals can be nowadays recorded unobtrusively by means of, for example, smartwatches and chest bands. These could provide an EMA and/or EMI platform with additional markers that more closely correlate to a person's affective state, and that can be used as input to the analysis performed [61]. Consistently, models can be automatically learned that continuously estimate the patient's affective state by extracting and analysing salient features of physiological signals [86]. For instance, electrodermal activity (EDA) and heart rate variability (HRV) have been extensively investigated as correlates of users' affective state, and they are considered non-invasive. They do not involve recording sensitive information (as opposed to, for example, cameras and acoustic signals), and associated sensors do not interfere with users' daily routines. Consistently, patient-specific models can be automatically learned that continuously estimate the patient's affective state by extracting and analysing salient features of physiological signals [86].

Unfortunately, the relation between physiological signals and affective states is not trivial and mixed results are discussed in the literature [87]. Building on recent advances of machine learning, recent studies obtained promising results by means of model personalisation for stress recognition [88] and deep learning for mood prediction [89] using a combination of behavioural and physiological markers in non-clinical populations. If thoroughly tested and consolidated through experimental validations in EMA settings, a model of this type could provide a finer-grained description of the evolution of the patient's disorder throughout a long-term study, compared to surveys that are usually filled in just a few times a day. It can be considered less obstructive to the patient's life because physiological data are recorded passively and do not require extra effort from the patient. Furthermore, in EMI settings, if the recognition algorithm detects that the patient is in a critical state, it can automatically trigger an intervention module associated with the platform or open a communication channel between the patient and his/her therapist. Alternatively, predictive models that combine information from physiological and behavioural signals to estimate the patient's future mood, stress level, and self-reported health (one or a few days in advance) can be automatically inferred [89]. After identifying a risk threshold, these models would make it possible to plan interventions (or involve the therapist) in advance, that is, before the patient's affective state reaches a critical state.

We should, however, recognize that the use of EMAs and EMIs has some limitations. These approaches are time-consuming and may be perceived as invasive by users. Patients are required to complete multiple assessments throughout a day, and protocols often last weeks. Moreover, people might not be willing to share personal information. Finally, in terms of more ecological validity, they may be advantageous for clinical purposes, but disadvantageous for research aims, because they imply less experimental control. Because the data are collected during everyday life and in naturalistic environments, it becomes hard or even impossible to have complete control over the setting, and, therefore, it is not possible to rule out the role of confounding variables. Nevertheless, due to the implementation of novel statistical procedures, a balance between research necessities and clinical utility could be achieved [90]. If this were the case in the near future, EMAs and EMIs would undoubtedly transform the field of mental health, greatly contributing to the bridging of science and practice [91,92].

Overall, this systematic review clearly shows the emergence of ecological assessment and intervention as a promising avenue for clinical psychology. The focus of the review was limited to a specific clinical population. Still, promising results have been already shown also regarding the application of EMA and EMI to anxiety disorders [93,94] and stress-related disorders [95,96], highlighting the potential of these tools to provide psychological support in daily life and to investigate symptom fluctuations across time. However, similar limitations and burning issues were also evidenced, including the need for more high-quality trials, the gap between the clinical and research field, and the importance of making EMAs and EMIs as engaging and tailored as possible. Altogether, there is evidence showing the feasibility and preliminary efficacy of these approaches, but much more research should be conducted before drawing definite conclusions.

Author Contributions: Conceptualization, D.C., J.F.-Á., A.G.P. and C.B.; methodology: D.C., J.F.-Á., M.S. and C.B.; writing—original draft preparation: D.C., J.F.-Á. and A.P.; writing—review and editing: C.B., A.G.P., P.C., M.K. and G.R.

Funding: This work was supported by the Marie Curie EF-ST AffecTech, approved at call H2020-MSCA-ITN-2016 (project reference: 722022).

Conflicts of Interest: The authors declare that no competing interests exist.

References

1. World Health Organization. *Depression and Other Common Mental Disorders: Global Health Estimates*; World Health Organization: Geneva, Switzerland, 2017; pp. 1–24.
2. Katon, W.; Ciechanowski, P. Impact of major depression on chronic medical illness. *J. Psychosom. Res.* **2002**, *53*, 859–863. [CrossRef]
3. Simon, G.E. Social and economic burden of mood disorders. *Biol. Psychiatry* **2003**, *54*, 208–215. [CrossRef]
4. Sullivan, L.E.; Fiellin, D.A.; O'Connor, P.G. The prevalence and impact of alcohol problems in major depression: A systematic review. *Am. J. Med.* **2005**, *118*, 330–341. [CrossRef] [PubMed]
5. Swendsen, J.D.; Merikangas, K.R. The comorbidity of depression and substance use disorders. *Clin. Psychol. Rev.* **2000**, *20*, 173–189. [CrossRef]
6. McConville, C.; Cooper, C. Mood variability and the intensity of depressive states. *Curr. Psychol.* **1996**, *14*, 329–338. [CrossRef]
7. Peeters, F.; Berkhof, J.; Delespaul, P.; Rottenberg, J.; Nicolson, N.A. Diurnal mood variation in major depressive disorder. *Emotion* **2006**, *6*, 383–391. [CrossRef] [PubMed]
8. Ben-Zeev, D.; Young, M.A.; Madsen, J.W. Retrospective recall of affect in clinically depressed individuals and controls. *Cogn. Emot.* **2009**. [CrossRef]
9. Chamberlain, S.R.; Sakakian, B.J. The neuropsychology of mood disorders. *Curr. Psychiatry Rep.* **2006**, *8*, 458–463. [CrossRef] [PubMed]
10. Möller, H.J.; von Zerssen, D. Self-rating procedures in the evaluation of antidepressants: Review of the literature and results of our studies. *Psychopathology* **1995**, *28*, 291–306. [CrossRef]
11. Gotlib, I.H.; Joormann, J. Cognition and Depression: Current Status and Future Directions. *Annu. Rev. Clin. Psychol.* **2010**, *6*, 285–312. [CrossRef]

12. Csikszentmihalyi, M.; Larson, R. Validity and Reliability of the Experience- Sampling Method. *J. Nerv. Ment. Dis.* **1987**, *175*, 526–536. [CrossRef] [PubMed]
13. Shiffman, S.; Stone, A.A.; Hufford, M.R. Ecological Momentary Assessment. *Annu. Rev. Clin. Psychol.* **2008**, *4*, 1–32. [CrossRef] [PubMed]
14. Stone, A.A.; Shiffman, S.; Atienza, A.A.; Nebeling, A. Historical roots and rationale of ecological momentary assessment (EMA). In *The Science of Real-Time Data Capture: Self-Reports in Health Research*; Oxford University Press: Oxford, MI, USA, 2007; pp. 3–10.
15. Aan het Rot, M.; Hogenelst, K.; Schoevers, R.A. Mood disorders in everyday life: A systematic review of experience sampling and ecological momentary assessment studies. *Clin. Psychol. Rev.* **2012**, *32*, 510–523. [CrossRef] [PubMed]
16. Ebner-Priemer, U.W.; Trull, T.J. Ecological momentary assessment of mood disorders and mood dysregulation. *Psychol. Assess.* **2009**, *21*, 463–475. [CrossRef] [PubMed]
17. Marzano, L.; Bardill, A.; Fields, B.; Herd, K.; Veale, D.; Grey, N.; Moran, P. The application of mHealth to mental health: Opportunities and challenges. *Lancet Psychiatry* **2015**, *2*, 942–948. [CrossRef]
18. Mohr, D.C.; Zhang, M.; Schueller, S.M. Personal Sensing: Understanding Mental Health Using Ubiquitous Sensors and Machine Learning. *Annu. Rev. Clin. Psychol.* **2017**, *13*, 23–47. [CrossRef] [PubMed]
19. van de Ven, P.; O'Brien, H.; Henriques, R.; Klein, M.; Msetfi, R.; Nelson, J.; Rocha, A.; Ruwaard, J.; O'Sullivan, D.; Riper, H. ULTEMAT: A mobile framework for smart ecological momentary assessments and interventions. *Internet Interv.* **2017**, *9*, 74–81. [CrossRef] [PubMed]
20. Henderson, C.; Evans-Lacko, S.; Thornicroft, G. Mental illness stigma, help seeking, and public health programs. *Am. J. Public Health* **2013**, *103*, 777–780. [CrossRef] [PubMed]
21. Kazdin, A.E.; Blase, S.L. Rebooting Psychotherapy Research and Practice to Reduce the Burden of Mental Illness. *Perspect. Psychol. Sci.* **2011**, *6*, 21–37. [CrossRef] [PubMed]
22. Heron, K.E.; Smyth, J.M. Ecological momentary interventions: Incorporating mobile technology into psychosocial and health behaviour treatments. *Br. J. Health Psychol.* **2010**, *15*, 1–39. [CrossRef] [PubMed]
23. Donker, T.; Petrie, K.; Proudfoot, J.; Clarke, J.; Birch, M.R.; Christensen, H. Smartphones for smarter delivery of mental health programs: A systematic review. *J. Med. Internet Res.* **2013**, *15*, e247. [CrossRef]
24. Cuijpers, P.; Donker, T.; Van Straten, A.; Li, J.; Andersson, G. Is guided self-help as effective as face-to-face psychotherapy for depression and anxiety disorders? A systematic review and meta-analysis of comparative outcome studies. *Psychol. Med.* **2010**, *40*, 1943–1957. [CrossRef] [PubMed]
25. Asada, H.H.; Shaltis, P.; Reisner, A.; Rhee, S.; Hutchinson, R.C. Mobile Monitoring with Wearable Photoplethysmographic Biosensors. *IEEE Eng. Med. Biol. Mag.* **2003**, *22*, 28–40. [CrossRef] [PubMed]
26. Torous, J.; Friedman, R.; Keshvan, M. Smartphone ownership and interest in mobile applications to monitor symptoms of mental health conditions. *J. Med. Internet Res.* **2014**, *16*. [CrossRef]
27. Moher, D.; Liberati, A.; Tetzlaff, J.; Altman, D.G.; PRISMA Group. Preferred reporting items for systematic reviews and meta analyses: The Prisma Statement. *PLoS Med.* **2009**, *6*, 1–15. [CrossRef] [PubMed]
28. Colombo, D.; Palacios, A.G.; Alvarez, J.F.; Patané, A.; Semonella, M.; Cipresso, P.; Kwiatkowska, M.; Riva, G.; Botella, C. Current state and future directions of technology-based ecological momentary assessments and interventions for major depressive disorder: Protocol for a systematic review. *Syst. Rev.* **2018**, *7*, 233. [CrossRef] [PubMed]
29. Delgadillo, J.; de Jong, K.; Lucock, M.; Lutz, W.; Rubel, J.; Gilbody, S.; Ali, S.; Aguirre, E.; Appleton, M.; Nevin, J.; et al. Feedback-informed treatment versus usual psychological treatment for depression and anxiety: A multisite, open-label, cluster randomised controlled trial. *Lancet Psychiatry* **2018**. [CrossRef]
30. Downs, S.H.; Black, N. The feasibility of creating a checklist for the assessment of the methodological quality both of randomised and non-randomised studies of health care interventions. *J. Epidemiol. Community Health* **1998**, *52*, 377–384. [CrossRef] [PubMed]
31. Conrad, A.; Wilhelm, F.H.; Roth, W.T.; Spiegel, D.; Taylor, C.B. Circadian affective, cardiopulmonary, and cortisol variability in depressed and nondepressed individuals at risk for cardiovascular disease. *J. Psychiatr. Res.* **2008**. [CrossRef]
32. Kim, J.; Nakamura, T.; Kikuchi, H.; Yoshiuchi, K.; Sasaki, T.; Yamamoto, Y. Covariation of Depressive Mood and Spontaneous Physical Activity in Major Depressive Disorder: Toward Continuous Monitoring of Depressive Mood. *IEEE J. Biomed. Heal. Inform.* **2015**, *19*, 1347–1355. [CrossRef]

33. Littlewood, D.L.; Kyle, S.D.; Carter, L.-A.; Peters, S.; Pratt, D.; Gooding, P. Short sleep duration and poor sleep quality predict next-day suicidal ideation: An ecological momentary assessment study. *Psychol. Med.* **2018**. [CrossRef] [PubMed]
34. Adams, Z.W.; McClure, E.A.; Gray, K.M.; Danielson, C.K.; Treiber, F.A.; Ruggiero, K.J. Mobile devices for the remote acquisition of physiological and behavioral biomarkers in psychiatric clinical research. *J. Psychiatr. Res.* **2017**. [CrossRef] [PubMed]
35. Ottaviani, C.; Shahabi, L.; Tarvainen, M.; Cook, I.; Abrams, M.; Shapiro, D. Cognitive, behavioral, and autonomic correlates of mind wandering and perseverative cognition in major depression. *Front. Neurosci.* **2015**. [CrossRef] [PubMed]
36. Booij, S.H.; Bos, E.H.; Bouwmans, M.E.J.; Van Faassen, M.; Kema, I.P.; Oldehinkel, A.J.; De Jonge, P. Cortisol and α-amylase secretion patterns between and within depressed and non-depressed individuals. *PLoS ONE* **2015**. [CrossRef] [PubMed]
37. Stavrakakis, N.; Booij, S.H.; Roest, A.M.; de Jonge, P.; Oldehinkel, A.J.; Bos, E.H. Temporal dynamics of physical activity and affect in depressed and nondepressed individuals. *Health Psychol.* **2015**, *34S*, 1268–1277. [CrossRef] [PubMed]
38. Bouwmans, M.E.J.; Oude Oosterik, N.A.M.; Bos, E.H.; de Groot, I.W.; Oldehinkel, A.J.; de Jonge, P. The Temporal Order of Changes in Physical Activity and Subjective Sleep in Depressed Versus Nondepressed Individuals: Findings From the MOOVD Study. *Behav. Sleep Med.* **2018**. [CrossRef] [PubMed]
39. Husky, M.M.; Gindre, C.; Mazure, C.M.; Brebant, C.; Nolen-Hoeksema, S.; Sanacora, G.; Swendsen, J. Computerized ambulatory monitoring in mood disorders: Feasibility, compliance, and reactivity. *Psychiatry Res.* **2010**. [CrossRef]
40. Schaffer, A.; Kreindler, D.; Reis, C.; Levitt, A.J. Use of Mental Health Telemetry to Enhance Identification and Predictive Value of Early Changes During Augmentation Treatment of Major Depression. *J. Clin. Psychopharmacol.* **2013**. [CrossRef] [PubMed]
41. Hung, S.; Li, M.-S.; Chen, Y.-L.; Chiang, J.-H.; Chen, Y.-Y.; Hung, G.C.-L. Smartphone-based ecological momentary assessment for Chinese patients with depression: An exploratory study in Taiwan. *Asian J. Psychiatr.* **2016**, *23*, 131–136. [CrossRef] [PubMed]
42. Stetler, C.; Dickerson, S.S.; Miller, G.E. Uncoupling of social zeitgebers and diurnal cortisol secretion in clinical depression. *Psychoneuroendocrinology* **2004**, *29*, 1250–1259. [CrossRef]
43. Stetler, C.; Miller, G.E. Blunted cortisol response to awakening in mild to moderate depression: Regulatory influences of sleep patterns and social contacts. *J. Abnorm. Psychol.* **2005**, *114*, 697–705. [CrossRef] [PubMed]
44. Huffziger, S.; Ebner-Priemer, U.; Zamoscik, V.; Reinhard, I.; Kirsch, P.; Kuehner, C. Effects of mood and rumination on cortisol levels in daily life: An ambulatory assessment study in remitted depressed patients and healthy controls. *Psychoneuroendocrinology* **2013**, *38*, 2258–2267. [CrossRef] [PubMed]
45. Booij, S.H.; Bos, E.H.; de Jonge, P.; Oldehinkel, A.J. The temporal dynamics of cortisol and affective states in depressed and non-depressed individuals. *Psychoneuroendocrinology* **2016**. [CrossRef] [PubMed]
46. Bower, B.; Bylsma, L.M.; Morris, B.H.; Rottenberg, J. Poor reported sleep quality predicts low positive affect in daily life among healthy and mood-disordered persons: Sleep quality and positive affect. *J. Sleep Res.* **2010**, *19*, 323–332. [CrossRef] [PubMed]
47. O'Leary, K.; Small, B.J.; Panaite, V.; Bylsma, L.M.; Rottenberg, J. Sleep quality in healthy and mood-disordered persons predicts daily life emotional reactivity. *Cogn. Emot.* **2017**, *31*, 435–443. [CrossRef] [PubMed]
48. Bouwmans, M.E.J.; Bos, E.H.; Hoenders, H.J.R.; Oldehinkel, A.J.; de Jonge, P. Sleep quality predicts positive and negative affect but not vice versa. An electronic diary study in depressed and healthy individuals. *J. Affect. Disord.* **2017**, *207*, 260–267. [CrossRef] [PubMed]
49. Bouwmans, M.E.J.; Beltz, A.M.; Bos, E.H.; Oldehinkel, A.J.; de Jonge, P.; Molenaar, P.C.M. The person-specific interplay of melatonin, affect, and fatigue in the context of sleep and depression. *Personal. Individ. Differ.* **2018**. [CrossRef]
50. Thompson, R.J.; Mata, J.; Jaeggi, S.M.; Buschkuehl, M.; Jonides, J.; Gotlib, I.H. The everyday emotional experience of adults with major depressive disorder: Examining emotional instability, inertia, and reactivity. *J. Abnorm. Psychol.* **2012**, *121*, 819–829. [CrossRef] [PubMed]
51. Putnam, K.M.; McSweeney, L.B. Depressive symptoms and baseline prefrontal EEG alpha activity: A study utilizing Ecological Momentary Assessment. *Biol. Psychol.* **2008**. [CrossRef]

52. Ruscio, A.M.; Gentes, E.L.; Jones, J.D.; Hallion, L.S.; Coleman, E.S.; Swendsen, J. Rumination Predicts Heightened Responding to Stressful Life Events in Major Depressive Disorder and Generalized Anxiety Disorder. *J. Abnorm. Psychol.* **2015**, *124*, 17–26. [CrossRef]
53. Kircanski, K.; Thompson, R.J.; Sorenson, J.; Sherdell, L.; Gotlib, I.H. The everyday dynamics of rumination and worry: Precipitant events and affective consequences. *Cogn. Emot.* **2018**, *32*, 1424–1436. [CrossRef] [PubMed]
54. Husky, M.M.; Mazure, C.M.; MacIejewski, P.K.; Swendsen, J.D. Past depression and gender interact to influence emotional reactivity to daily life stress. *Cognit. Ther. Res.* **2009**, *33*, 264–271. [CrossRef]
55. Bylsma, L.M.; Taylor-Clift, A.; Rottenberg, J. Emotional reactivity to daily events in major and minor depression. *J. Abnorm. Psychol.* **2011**. [CrossRef]
56. Kohling, J.; Moessner, M.; Ehrenthal, J.C.; Bauer, S.; Cierpka, M.; Kammerer, A.; Schauenburg, H.; Dinger, U.; Köhling, J.; Moessner, M.; et al. Affective Instability and Reactivity in Depressed Patients With and Without Borderline Pathology. *J. Personal. Disord.* **2015**, *30*, 1–20. [CrossRef] [PubMed]
57. Slofstra, C.; Nauta, M.H.; Holmes, E.A.; Bos, E.H.; Wichers, M.; Batalas, N.; Klein, N.S.; Bockting, C.L.H. Exploring the relation between visual mental imagery and affect in the daily life of previously depressed and never depressed individuals. *Cogn. Emot.* **2018**, *32*, 1131–1138. [CrossRef] [PubMed]
58. Hepp, J.; Lane, S.P.; Carpenter, R.W.; Niedtfeld, I.; Brown, W.C.; Trull, T.J. Interpersonal Problems and Negative Affect in Borderline Personality and Depressive Disorders in Daily Life. *Clin. Psychol. Sci.* **2017**. [CrossRef] [PubMed]
59. Quilty, L.C.; Watson, C.; Toneatto, T.; Bagby, R.M. A Prospective Investigation of Affect, the Desire to Gamble, Gambling Motivations and Gambling Behavior in the Mood Disorders. *J. Gambl. Stud.* **2017**. [CrossRef] [PubMed]
60. Fisher, A.J.; Reeves, J.W.; Lawyer, G.; Medaglia, J.D.; Rubel, J.A. Exploring the idiographic dynamics of mood and anxiety via network analysis. *J. Abnorm. Psychol.* **2017**. [CrossRef] [PubMed]
61. Burns, M.N.; Begale, M.; Duffecy, J.; Gergle, D.; Karr, C.J.; Giangrande, E.; Mohr, D.C. Harnessing context sensing to develop a mobile intervention for depression. *J. Med. Internet Res.* **2011**, *13*. [CrossRef]
62. Kramer, I.; Simons, C.J.P.; Hartmann, J.A.; Menne-Lothmann, C.; Viechtbauer, W.; Peeters, F.; Schruers, K.; van Bemmel, A.L.; Myin-Germeys, I.; Delespaul, P.; et al. A therapeutic application of the experience sampling method in the treatment of depression: A randomized controlled trial. *World Psychiatry* **2014**, *13*, 68–77. [CrossRef]
63. Simons, C.J.P.; Hartmann, J.A.; Kramer, I.; Menne-Lothmann, C.; Höhn, P.; van Bemmel, A.L.; Myin-Germeys, I.; Delespaul, P.; van Os, J.; Wichers, M. Effects of momentary self-monitoring on empowerment in a randomized controlled trial in patients with depression. *Eur. Psychiatry* **2015**. [CrossRef]
64. Hartmann, J.A.; Wichers, M.; Menne-Lothmann, C.; Kramer, I.; Viechtbauer, W.; Peeters, F.; Schruers, K.R.J.; Van Bemmel, A.L.; Myin-Germeys, I.; Delespaul, P.; et al. Experience sampling-based personalized feedback and Positive affect: A randomized controlled trial in depressed patients. *PLoS ONE* **2015**, *10*. [CrossRef] [PubMed]
65. Mohr, D.C.; Stiles-Shields, C.; Brenner, C.; Palac, H.; Montague, E.; Kaiser, S.M.; Carty-Fickes, E.; Duffecy, J. MedLink: A Mobile Intervention to Address Failure Points in the Treatment of Depression in General Medicine. *Int. Conf. Pervasive Comput. Technol. Healthc.* **2015**, *2015*, 100–107. [PubMed]
66. Burton, C.; Szentagotai Tatar, A.; McKinstry, B.; Matheson, C.; Matu, S.; Moldovan, R.; Macnab, M.; Farrow, E.; David, D.; Pagliari, C.; et al. Pilot randomised controlled trial of Help4Mood, an embodied virtual agent-based system to support treatment of depression. *J. Telemed. Telecare* **2016**, *22*, 348–355. [CrossRef]
67. Snippe, E.; Simons, C.J.P.; Hartmann, J.A.; Menne-Lothmann, C.; Kramer, I.; Booij, S.H.; Viechtbauer, W.; Delespaul, P.; Myin-Germeys, I.; Wichers, M. Change in daily life behaviors and depression: Within-person and between-person associations. *Health Psychol.* **2016**, *35*, 433–441. [CrossRef] [PubMed]
68. Widdershoven, R.L.A.; Wichers, M.; Kuppens, P.; Hartmann, J.A.; Menne-Lothmann, C.; Simons, C.J.P.; Bastiaansen, J.A. Effect of self-monitoring through experience sampling on emotion differentiation in depression. *J. Affect. Disord.* **2019**. [CrossRef] [PubMed]
69. Torous, J.; Staples, P.; Shanahan, M.; Lin, C.; Peck, P.; Keshavan, M.; Onnela, J.-P. Utilizing a Personal Smartphone Custom App to Assess the Patient Health Questionnaire-9 (PHQ-9) Depressive Symptoms in Patients With Major Depressive Disorder. *JMIR Ment. Health* **2015**, *2*, e8. [CrossRef]

70. Nilsen, W.J.; Pavel, M. Moving behavioral theories into the 21st century: Technological advancements for improving quality of life. *IEEE Pulse* **2013**, *4*, 25–28. [CrossRef]
71. Ericsson Consumer Lab Eurupe Ericsson Mobility Report Appendix. *Ericsson Mobil. Rep.* **2015**, 1–8. [CrossRef]
72. Ben-Zeev, D.; Davis, K.E.; Kaiser, S.; Krzsos, I.; Drake, R.E. Mobile technologies among people with serious mental illness: Opportunities for future services. *Adm. Policy Ment. Health* **2013**, *40*, 340–343. [CrossRef]
73. Colombo, D.; Cipresso, P.; Fernández Alvarez, J.; Garcia Palacios, A.; Riva, G.; Botella, C. An Overview of Factors Associated with Adherence and Dropout to Ecological Momentary Assessments in Depression. *Annu. Rev. CyberTherapy Telemed.* **2018**, in press.
74. Karyotaki, E.; Kleiboer, A.; Smit, F.; Turner, D.T.; Pastor, A.M.; Andersson, G.; Berger, T.; Botella, C.; Breton, J.M.; Carlbring, P.; et al. Predictors of treatment dropout in self-guided web-based interventions for depression: An "individual patient data" meta-analysis. *Psychol. Med.* **2015**. [CrossRef] [PubMed]
75. Kuppens, P.; Verduyn, P. Emotion dynamics. *Curr. Opin. Psychol.* **2017**, *17*, 22–26. [CrossRef] [PubMed]
76. Boswell, J.F.; Kraus, D.R.; Miller, S.D.; Lambert, M.J. Implementing routine outcome monitoring in clinical practice: Benefits, challenges, and solutions. *Psychother. Res.* **2015**. [CrossRef] [PubMed]
77. Mikus, A.; Hoogendoorn, M.; Rocha, A.; Gama, J.; Ruwaard, J.; Riper, H. Predicting short term mood developments among depressed patients using adherence and ecological momentary assessment data. *Internet Interv.* **2018**, *12*, 105–110. [CrossRef]
78. Nuij, C.; van Ballegooijen, W.; Ruwaard, J.; de Beurs, D.; Mokkenstorm, J.; van Duijn, E.; de Winter, R.F.P.; O'Connor, R.C.; Smit, J.H.; Riper, H.; et al. Smartphone-based safety planning and self-monitoring for suicidal patients: Rationale and study protocol of the CASPAR (Continuous Assessment for Suicide Prevention And Research) study. *Internet Interv.* **2018**. [CrossRef] [PubMed]
79. Saranummi, N.; Spruijt-Metz, D.; Intille, S.S.; Korhonen, I.; Nilsen, W.J.; Pavel, M. Moving the science of behavioral change into the 21st century: Part 2. *IEEE Pulse* **2013**, *4*, 32–33. [CrossRef] [PubMed]
80. Brown, M.; O'Neill, N.; van Woerden, H.; Eslambolchilar, P.; Jones, M.; John, A. Gamification and Adherence to Web-Based Mental Health Interventions: A Systematic Review. *JMIR Ment. Health* **2016**, *3*, e39. [CrossRef] [PubMed]
81. Majumder, S.; Mondal, T.; Deen, M. Wearable Sensors for Remote Health Monitoring. *Sensors* **2017**, *17*, 130. [CrossRef] [PubMed]
82. Aziz, O.; Atallah, L.; Lo, B.; ElHelw, M.; Wang, L.; Yang, G.Z.; Darzi, A. A pervasive body sensor network for measuring postoperative recovery at home. *Surg. Innov.* **2007**. [CrossRef]
83. Patel, S.; Park, H.; Bonato, P.; Chan, L.; Rodgers, M. A review of wearable sensors and systems with application in rehabilitation. *J. Neuroeng. Rehabil.* **2012**, *9*, 21. [CrossRef]
84. Ohta, S.; Nakamoto, H.; Shinagawa, Y.; Tanikawa, T. A health monitoring system for elderly people living alone. *J. Telemed. Telecare* **2002**. [CrossRef]
85. Seppälä, J.; De Vita, I.; Jämsä, T.; Miettunen, J.; Isohanni, M.; Rubinstein, K.; Feldman, Y.; Grasa, E.; Corripio, I.; Berdun, J.; et al. Mobile Phone and Wearable Sensor-Based mHealth Approaches for Psychiatric Disorders and Symptoms: Systematic Review. *JMIR Ment. Health* **2019**, *6*, e9819. [CrossRef]
86. Lisetti, C.L.; Nasoz, F. Using noninvasive wearable computers to recognize human emotions from physiological signals. *EURASIP J. Appl. Signal Process.* **2004**, *2004*, 1672–1687. [CrossRef]
87. Choi, K.H.; Kim, J.; Kwon, O.S.; Kim, M.J.; Ryu, Y.H.; Park, J.E. Is heart rate variability (HRV) an adequate tool for evaluating human emotions? A focus on the use of the International Affective Picture System (IAPS). *Psychiatry Res.* **2017**. [CrossRef]
88. Kocielnik, R.; Sidorova, N.; Maggi, F.M.; Ouwerkerk, M.; Westerink, J.H.D.M. Smart technologies for long-term stress monitoring at work. In Proceedings of the CBMS 2013—26th IEEE International Symposium on Computer-Based Medical Systems, Porto, Portugal, 20–22 June 2013.
89. Shen, N.; Levitan, M.-J.; Johnson, A.; Bender, J.L.; Hamilton-Page, M.; Jadad, A.A.R.; Wiljer, D. Finding a Depression App: A Review and Content Analysis of the Depression App Marketplace. *JMIR Mhealth Uhealth* **2015**, *3*, e16. [CrossRef]
90. Lin, X.; Mermelstein, R.J.; Hedeker, D. A 3-level Bayesian mixed effects location scale model with an application to ecological momentary assessment data. *Stat. Med.* **2018**. [CrossRef]
91. Goldfried, M.R. The future of psychotherapy integration: Closing the gap between research and practice. *J. Psychother. Integr.* **2010**, *20*, 386–396. [CrossRef]

92. Fernández-Álvarez, J.; Fernández-Álvarez, H.; Castonguay, L.G. Summarizing Novel Efforts to Integrate Practice and Research from a Practice Oriented Research Perspective. *Rev. Argent. Clín. Psicol.* **2018**, *27*, 353–362. [CrossRef]
93. Walz, L.C.; Nauta, M.H.; aan het Rot, M. Experience sampling and ecological momentary assessment for studying the daily lives of patients with anxiety disorders: A systematic review. *J. Anxiety Disord.* **2014**, *28*, 925–937. [CrossRef]
94. Schueller, S.M.; Aguilera, A.; Mohr, D.C. Ecological momentary interventions for depression and anxiety. *Depress. Anxiety* **2017**, *34*, 540–545. [CrossRef] [PubMed]
95. Yoshiuchi, K.; Yamamoto, Y.; Akabayashi, A. Application of ecological momentary assessment in stress-related diseases. *Biopsychosoc. Med.* **2008**, *2*, 13. [CrossRef] [PubMed]
96. Gee, B.L.; Griffiths, K.M.; Gulliver, A. Effectiveness of mobile technologies delivering Ecological Momentary Interventions for stress and anxiety: A systematic review. *J. Am. Med. Inform. Assoc.* **2016**. [CrossRef]

Journal of
Clinical Medicine

MDPI

Article

Experienced Burden of and Adherence to Smartphone-Based Ecological Momentary Assessment in Persons with Affective Disorders

Claire R. van Genugten [1,2,*], Josien Schuurmans [1,2], Femke Lamers [2], Harriëtte Riese [3], Brenda W. J. H. Penninx [1,2], Robert A. Schoevers [3], Heleen M. Riper [1,2,4,5] and Johannes H. Smit [1,2]

1 Department of Research and Innovation, GGZ inGeest, Specialized Mental Health Care, 1081 Amsterdam, The Netherlands; j.schuurmans@ggzingeest.nl (J.S.); b.penninx@amsterdamumc.nl (B.W.J.H.P.); h.riper@vu.nl (H.M.R.); jh.smit@ggzingeest.nl (J.H.S.)

2 Department of Psychiatry, Amsterdam Public Health Research Institute, Amsterdam UMC, Vrije Universiteit, 1081 Amsterdam, The Netherlands; f.lamers@ggzingeest.nl

3 Interdisciplinary Centre for Psychopathology and Emotion Regulation, Department of Psychiatry, University Medical Centre Groningen, University of Groningen, 9713 Groningen, The Netherlands; h.riese@umcg.nl (H.R.); r.a.schoevers@umcg.nl (R.A.S.)

4 Department of Clinical, Neuro and Developmental Psychology, Clinical Psychology Section, Vrije Universiteit Amsterdam and the Amsterdam Public Health Research Institute, 1081 Amsterdam, The Netherlands

5 Institute of Telepsychiatry, University of Southern Denmark, 5000 Odense, Denmark

* Correspondence: c.genugten@ggzingeest.nl; Tel.: +31-(0)207884625

Received: 28 December 2019; Accepted: 21 January 2020; Published: 23 January 2020

Abstract: (1) Background: The use of smartphone-based ecological momentary assessment (EMA) questionnaires in affective disorder research has rapidly increased. Though, a thorough understanding of experienced burden of and adherence to EMA is crucial in determining the usefulness of EMA. (2) Methods: Persons with current affective disorders (n = 100), remitted persons (n = 190), and healthy controls (n = 94) participated in a smartphone-based EMA two-week monitoring period. Our primary outcomes were (momentary) perceived burden of and adherence to EMA. (3) Results: In the whole sample, lower positive and higher negative affect were associated with slightly higher levels of perceived momentary burden (B = −0.23 [95%CI = −0.27–0.19], B = 0.30 [95%CI = 0.24–0.37], respectively). The persons with current affective disorders reported slightly higher levels of experienced momentary burden (Mdn = 1.98 [IQR = 1.28–2.57]), than the remitted persons (Mdn = 1.64 [IQR = 1.11–2.24]) and healthy controls (Mdn = 1.28 [IQR = 1.04–1.92]). Nevertheless, the persons with current affective disorders still showed very high adherence rates (Mdn = 94.3% [IQR = 87.9–97.1]), at rates on a par with the remitted persons (Mdn = 94.3% [IQR = 90.0–97.1]) and healthy controls (Mdn = 94.3% [IQR = 90.0–98.6]). (4) Discussion: Frequent momentary questionnaires of mental well-being are slightly more burdensome to the persons with current affective disorders, but this does not seem to have a negative impact on adherence. Their high rate of adherence to EMA—which was similar to that in remitted persons and healthy controls —suggests that it is feasible to apply (short-duration) EMA.

Keywords: affective disorders; depression; anxiety disorders; ecological momentary assessment; burden; adherence

1. Background

In recent decades, we have witnessed a surge in research acknowledging the importance of real-life context and diurnal variation of affective states in persons with affective disorders [1–4]. Ecological momentary assessment (EMA) is a valuable addition to the traditional methods of studying these dynamics [5–8]. EMA questionnaires were initially administered via paper-and-pencil diaries. Nowadays, online tools or apps on devices such as mobile telephones are designed to capture momentary ratings. With EMA, participants are asked to self-report information on their momentary affect throughout the day in natural settings [7–9], rather than recalling and summarizing their affect within a certain time interval (e.g., last week/month), as is done in retrospective questionnaires [9].

Advocates of EMA argue that assessing affective states more frequently is a more appropriate way to measure affect dynamics, as retrospective distortions are minimized [6,10–13]. EMA questionnaires provide us with the essential information that needs to be measured in order to generate insights in the temporal variability of anxiety and mood symptoms, the importance of real-life context, phenomenology, and the interrelatedness of symptoms [14–16]. These nuances are hard to capture when using traditional retrospective questionnaires, for the reasons mentioned above.

Measuring affect more frequently means that persons are repeatedly asked to provide information on their own mental well-being. However, since symptoms such as a lack of motivation to act and problems concentrating are core features of the clinical presentation of depression [17,18], adhering to these repeated questionnaires is not self-evident for persons with affective disorders. Also, repeatedly assessing affective states in persons who suffer from a persistently negative mood might lead to high levels of perceived burden. Nevertheless, systematic reviews showed encouraging results regarding the burden experienced and adherence rates by persons with affective disorders [8,14,15]. However, studies only investigated burden in terms of a reflection on the whole monitoring period; momentary burden, e.g., perceived burden at the moment of measuring, was not taken into account in any of these studies. Moreover, the majority of studies reporting on adherence rates used EMA methods such as paper-and-pencil diaries and personal digital assistants (PDAs) instead of smartphone-based EMA questionnaires. Adherence to smartphone-based EMA might differ from other EMA methods; nowadays the use of telephones is incorporated in the daily lives of many persons, as opposed to paper-and-pencil diaries and PDAs that were distributed for study-purposes only. A better understanding of experiences of users is crucial when considering the usefulness of smartphone-based EMA questionnaires for persons with affective disorders.

The aim of this study was to explore perceived burden and adherence to smartphone-based EMA questionnaires in persons with affective disorders sampled from the Ecological Momentary Assessment (EMA) and Actigraphy sub-study (NESDA-EMAA) [19,20]. As well as persons with affective disorders, the cohort also included remitted persons and healthy controls. All (n = 384) participated in an interview, including a clinical assessment and an intensive two-week smartphone-based EMA monitoring period with five EMA questionnaires a day. Due to this design, we were able to make a direct comparison in adherence and perceived burden between the persons with current affective disorders and the other two groups in a single cohort.

2. Methods

2.1. Study Design and Participants

The participants of the Ecological Momentary Assessment (EMA) and Actigraphy sub-study (NESDA-EMAA) were selected from the Netherlands Study of Depression and Anxiety (NESDA). In brief, NESDA is an ongoing longitudinal multi-site naturalistic cohort study which aims to examine the biological, social, and psychological factors contributing to the long-term course of depressive and anxiety disorders [21]. NESDA participants were initially recruited for the baseline measurement between 2004 and 2007 (n = 2981) and were invited for a fifth interview on the occasion of the nine-year follow-up measurement (Wave 6; 2014-2017; n = 1776). At Wave 6, siblings (n = 367) of a subsample of NESDA participants were also recruited and included in the NESDA cohort.

Wave 6 comprised a large number of measurements, administered by trained research staff. These included a structured clinical diagnostic interview. After measurement, the participants were invited to join the NESDA-EMAA. For the NESDA-EMAA we invited NESDA participants who participated in at least two of the previous waves, consented to be approached for the NESDA-EMAA, participated in the interview no more than 31 days prior starting with the EMA questionnaires, were familiar with smartphone use and willing to wear a wrist-worn actigraphy device. Siblings were invited if they did not meet the criteria of a current or past diagnosis of depressive and/or anxiety disorder or other severe psychiatric disorder [19,20]. A flowchart showing the enrolment processes is given in Figure 1.

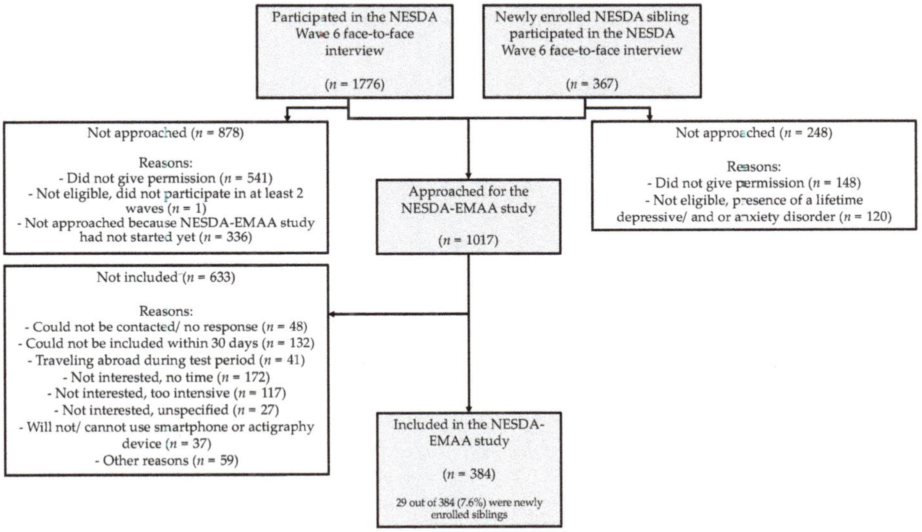

Figure 1. Flowchart of the Ecological Momentary Assessment (EMA) and Actigraphy sub-study (NESDA-EMAA).

This resulted in a sample of 384 included participants (of whom 29 were newly enrolled siblings). The sample was divided into three groups: 1) a group with at least one current affective disorder (n = 100) (i.e., persons who met the criteria for a depressive or anxiety disorder in the past six months, per to the Diagnostic and Statistical Manual of Mental Disorders, Fourth Edition, Text Revision (DSM-IV-TR) criteria); 2) a group with an affective disorder in remission (n = 190) (persons with a life-time diagnosis of depressive and/or anxiety disorder, but who did not meet DSM-IV-TR criteria in the past six months); and 3) a healthy control group (n = 94) (persons with no lifetime history of psychiatric disorders). The in- and exclusion criteria are described in more detail elsewhere [19,20].

The study was carried out in accordance with the latest version of the Declaration of Helsinki. The Ethical Review Board of VU University Medical Centre Amsterdam and the local review boards of the participating centres provided ethical approval and all participants provided written consent. The NESDA and the NESDA-EMAA are described in more detail elsewhere [19–21].

2.2. Smartphone-Based Ecological Momentary Assessment Protocol

All the NESDA-EMAA participants were invited to conduct five EMA questionnaires a day for 14 days. These were conducted during the day, using a time-based sampling protocol with fixed time intervals of three hours. The questionnaires were in the form of self-reported answers with a maximum of 31 questions, focusing on momentary affective states, as well as a number of additional items such as hours of sleep since the last questionnaire. Data were collected via smartphones; at an appointed time, the participants received an invitation by text message to conduct and submit the questionnaire. Participants were instructed to complete the questionnaire as soon as possible after receiving the text message, preferably within 15 minutes, but at least within 60 minutes. After completing the questionnaires, the participant's answers were saved automatically to the secured web-based server (RoQua) [22].

In addition to the automatic reminder, several measures were taken to motivate the participants and to provide support when needed. Research assistants called them on at least two separate occasions: one day and one week after the moment they started with the questionnaires. Additionally, participants received a gift voucher worth €20 and a personalized report of their EMA questionnaires afterwards.

2.3. Measurements

2.3.1. Baseline Characteristics

Basic demographics and clinical characteristics were requested during the Wave 6 measurement. We obtained information about age, gender, and educational level through standard questions. Number of current weekly working hours was assessed by the use of the Treatment Inventory of Costs in Patients with psychiatric disorders (TiC-P) [23]. Presence of lifetime and/or current depressive (dysthymia and major depressive disorder) and anxiety disorders (social anxiety disorder, panic disorder with or without agoraphobia, agoraphobia, and generalized anxiety disorder) was defined according to DSM-IV criteria [24]. Diagnoses were established using the Composite International Diagnostic Interview (CIDI Version 2.1) [25]. This has high validity for the assessment of mental disorders [26].

2.3.2. Momentary Affective States

Momentary affective states were measured repeatedly through the daily EMA questionnaires. The participants provided information about their mental well-being by completing a thirteen-item questionnaire. Twelve of these items were derived from the affect-questionnaire in the Uncovering Positive Potential of Emotional Reactivity (UPPER) study [27]. For this study we added a thirteenth item on feelings of anxiety. The list included seven items covering the negative affective state, whilst the other six covered the positive state. The negative affect items (At this moment I feel upset, irritated, listless/apathic, down, nervous, bored, anxious) were averaged to form a negative affect (NA) subscale and the positive affect ones (At this moment I feel satisfied, relaxed, cheerful, energetic, enthusiastic, calm) were averaged to form a positive affect (PA) subscale. The items were rated on seven-point Likert scales (1 = not at all, 4 = moderate, 7 = very); higher scores meant respectively higher levels of negative and positive affect.

2.4. Outcomes

2.4.1. Momentary Burden

Experienced burden as a result of the daily EMA questionnaires was one of the main outcomes of this study. We assessed momentary burden; participants were asked about their experienced burden as a result of the EMA questionnaire itself. They did so by answering the following standard question "How disturbing is filling out a questionnaire right now?". The question was rated on a seven-point Likert scale (1 = not at all, 4 = moderate, 7 = very).

2.4.2. Experienced Burden Over the Whole Monitoring Period

We also assessed the participants' overall experience. Immediately after the last daily EMA questionnaire, participants received a text message with a link to an addendum questionnaire, which included four items to evaluate experienced burden over the whole EMA monitoring period. Questions about the study duration; the number of questions; assessment frequency; and overall experience were rated on a seven-point Likert scale (1 = not at all, 4 = moderate, 7 = very). The average of these four items represented the evaluation score (sum possibilities ranging from 1 to 7). The four items showed excellent internal consistency in this sample (Cronbach's $\alpha = 0.924$).

2.4.3. Adherence to the Daily EMA Questionnaires

The other main outcome of this study was adherence to the daily EMA questionnaires. This was calculated by counting the percentage of completed EMA questionnaires out of the total of 70 each participant was invited to undertake. Moreover, at the last EMA questionnaire participants were asked to report their main reasons for missing a questionnaire, if they had done so. Possible reasons listed in the questionnaire were: being busy with an activity; no network connection; being asleep; technical problems; not hearing the smartphone; not bringing the smartphone; could not making themselves do it; and "other" reasons. The participants were allowed to select more than one reason. In addition, we counted the absolute number of omissions due to technical issues.

2.5. Statistical Analyses

We calculated descriptive statistics for the majority of our variables. Because data appeared to be non-normally distributed based on Kolmogorov–Smirnov tests, we report the median (Mdn) and the interquartile range (IQR) for the continuous variables. Differences between the three diagnosis groups in terms of demographic characteristics, absolute number of uploaded assessments, the retrospective evaluation sum-score, and reported reasons for missing assessments were analyzed; for this we used Kruskall–Wallis tests, Bonferroni-adjusted Mann–Whitney tests, Pearson chi-square tests, and likelihood ratio tests as appropriate.

To analyze the EMA data, we conducted several tests. We looked at whether the groups differed in respect of mean momentary burden as reported through the daily EMA questionnaires. In order to do this, we first calculated the person-mean of this variable by averaging the scores across the participants' EMA questionnaires. We then compared the averages of the person-mean scores for the three diagnosis groups using a Kruskall–Wallis test and conducted pairwise comparisons using Bonferroni-adjusted Mann–Whitney tests. In addition, we produced a number of generalized estimated equation (GEE) models for the overall sample. We chose GEE models because EMA data have a hierarchical structure; this type of model adjusts for dependency of repeated measures within one participant and can handle non-normally distributed data. GEE models are also suitable for dealing with missing data; it is not required to exclude participants with missing questionnaires, nor should missing questionnaires be imputed beforehand. A more detailed description about GEE models is described in detail elsewhere [28,29]. We used the GEE models to analyze the association between positive and negative affect on the one hand, and momentary burden as a result of the measurement itself on the other. The variables diagnosis group, gender, age, weekly working hours, and educational level were separately added to the GEE models as independent variables to check for possible confounding. Next, the variables were added as interaction terms to the model to check for possible effect modification. A GEE model was also used to analyze the stability of the reported levels of momentary burden across the EMA questionnaires. To see whether levels of burden changed as the study period progressed, we added the variable time to the unadjusted model. All analyses were carried out using SPSS (version 25.0) and two-sides p values < 0.05 were considered significant ($p < 0.017$ after Bonferroni correction).

3. Results

3.1. Sample Characteristics

Table 1 shows the demographic and clinical characteristics that were assessed across the three diagnosis groups. In the overall sample, 67.0% (238 out of 384) of the participants were female, the median age was 51.0 years (IQR = 38.00–61.00), the average of weekly working hours was 20

(IQR = 0.00–35.5), and most individuals had intermediate (50.3% [193 out of 384]) or high (46.4% [178 out of 384]) education. In general, a considerable number of persons with current affective disorder and remitted persons suffered multiple affective disorder at the time of the EMA questionnaires or in their history, respectively. In total, 39.0% (39 out of 100) of the persons with current affective disorders suffered from more than one affective disorder (range 2–7) at the time of the EMA questionnaires. In the group of persons with remitted persons, 66.3% (126 out of 190) suffered from more than one affective disorder (range 2–7), in parallel or in sequence, in their life span.

Table 1. Demographics of the study sample.

	Persons with Current Affective Disorder(S) Persons (n = 100)	Remitted Persons (n = 190)	Healthy Controls (n = 94)	Total (n = 384)	Test Value	p Value
Demographic characteristics						
Age	50.5 (41.5–59.0)	48.5 (36.0–61.0)	54.0 (4.0–62.0)	51.0 (38.0–61.0)	H(2) = 4.25	0.12
Gender						
Female	64 (64.0)	132 (69.5)	51 (54.3)	238 (67.0)	$\chi^2(2) = 6.35$	0.04
Male	36 (36.0)	58 (30.5)	43 (45.7)	117 (33.0)		
Educational level						
Basic	8 (8.0)	4 (2.1)	1 (1.1)	13 (3.4)	$\chi^2(4) = 14.51$	0.01
Intermediate	49 (49.0)	106 (55.8)	38 (40.4)	193 (50.3)		
High	43 (43.0)	80 (42.1)	55 (58.5)	178 (46.4)		
Working hours (a week)	10.0 (0.0–32.0)	20.0 (0.0–32.0)	30.0 (0.0–37.0)	20.0 (0.0–35.5)	H(2) = 10.22	0.01
DSM-IV-R Diagnosis	**Current**	**Lifetime**				
One more or anxiety disorder	71(71.0)	142 (74.7)				
One or more depressive disorder	61 (61.0)	163 (85.8)				
Generalized anxiety disorder	12 (12.0)	69 (36.3)				
Social phobia	35 (35.0)	86 (45.3)				
Panic disorder with agoraphobia	6 (6.0)	41 (21.6)				
Panic disorder without agoraphobia	13 (13.0)	31 (16.3)				
Agoraphobia	22 (22.0)	32 (16.8)				
Major depressive disorder	57 (57.0)	160 (84.2)				
Dysthymia	15 (15.0)	52 (27.4)				
Number of affective disorders*	**Current**	**Lifetime**				
1	61 (61.0)	64 (33.7)				
2	23 (23.0)	45 (23.7)				
3	12 (12.0)	39 (20.5)				
4	3 (3.0)	22 (11.6)				
5	1 (1.0)	10 (5.3)				
6	0 (0.0)	8 (4.2)				
7	0 (0.0)	2 (1.1)				

Note: Data are n (%), mean (SD) or median (IQR). Kruskall–Wallis, Pearson's chi-square and likelihood ratio tests were used as appropriate. * Affective disorders include depressive disorders (major depressive disorder, dysthymia) and anxiety disorders (social anxiety disorder, panic disorder with or without agoraphobia, agoraphobia, and generalized anxiety disorder).

3.2. Burden

3.2.1. Person-Mean Momentary Burden

To examine perceived burden as a result of the daily EMA questionnaires, we looked at momentary burden and at an evaluation of experienced burden over the whole two-week EMA monitoring period. Figure 2 shows the distribution of the person-means of the momentary burden in the three diagnosis groups. Tests showed a significant difference between the three groups (H[2] = 17.31, $p < 0.0001$). Subsequent, Bonferroni-corrected pairwise comparisons showed that, on average, the person-means of momentary burden reported by the persons with current affective disorders (Mdn = 1.98, IQR = 1.28–2.57) were significantly higher than in both the remitted persons (Mdn = 1.64, IQR = 1.11–2.24; U = 7229.50, p = 0.01) and the healthy controls (Mdn = 1.28, IQR = 1.04–1.92; U = 3098.50, $p < 0.0001$).

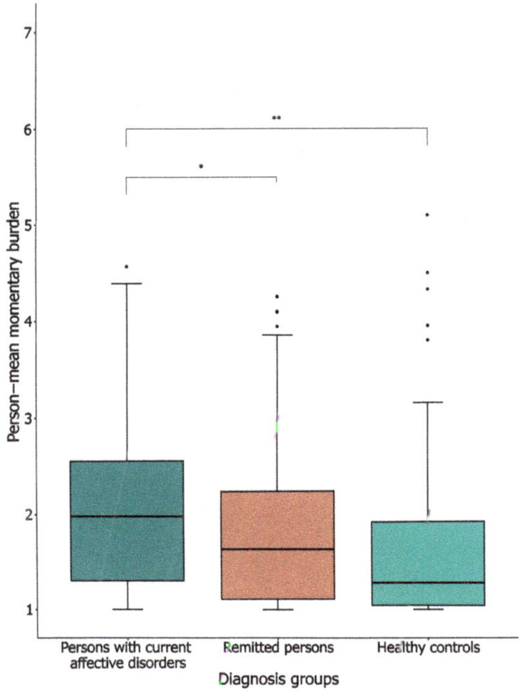

Figure 2. Person-mean momentary burden as reported on the EMA measures. Note: Value labels: 1 = 'No burden'; 4 = 'Moderate burden'; 7 = 'High burden'. Thick black line shows the median, error bars show the interquartile range (IQR), whiskers show +/−1.5 IQR, ● = outlier, deviates by ≥ 1.5× IQR, * = significant at $p < 0.017$ (Bonferroni-adjustment), and ** = significant at $p < 0.0001$. 3.3. Adherence to the daily EMA questionnaires.

3.2.2. Association Between Affective States and Momentary Burden

Table 2 shows the results of the unadjusted and adjusted GEE analyses, calculated over the whole sample (with a total of 24,537 completed EMA questionnaires). First, we found a significant negative association between positive affect and momentary burden (B = −0.23, 95%CI = −0.27–0.19, $p < 0.0001$), and a significant positive association between negative affect and momentary burden (B = 0.30, 95%CI = −0.24–0.37, $p < 0.0001$). These coefficients indicate that a score of 1.00 higher on the PA scale (range 1–7) is associated with −0.23 points less reported burden (range 1–7) and 1.00 point higher on the NA scale (range 1–7) is associated with 0.30 higher reported burden (range 1–7). Hereafter, in both analyses, the variables diagnosis group, weekly working hours, gender, age, and educational background were separately added to the model to check for possible confounding. None of these variables were considered a confounder. In addition, in neither analysis did we find significant interaction between these five covariates on the one hand, and positive or negative affect on the other. Next, regards the stability of momentary burden (i.e., to see whether levels of burden changed as the study period progressed); we found that the strength of the association between reported levels of burden as a result of the questionnaires did not change significantly over time (B = 0.00, 95%CI = 0.00-0.00, $p = 0.09$). To conclude, these results indicate that lower positive affect and higher negative affect were associated with slightly higher levels of momentary burden, regardless of the presence of a current affective disorder, number of weekly working hours, age, gender, and educational background. Also, reported level of burden remained stable over time across the whole sample.

Table 2. Association between momentary burden, affective scales and time.

		Regression Coefficient (Standard Error)	95%CI	Test Value	p Value
Positive affect and momentary burden					
Positive affect (PA) *		−0.23 (0.02)	−0.27–0.19	$\chi^2(1) = 130.77$	<0.0001
+ diagnosis groups		−0.22 (0.02)	−0.26–0.18	$\chi^2(1) = 114.36$	<0.0001
+ weekly working hours		−0.23 (0.02)	−0.27–0.19	$\chi^2(1) = 133.58$	<0.0001
+ gender		−0.23 (0.02)	−0.27–0.19	$\chi^2(1) = 131.38$	<0.0001
+ age		−0.23 (0.02)	−0.27–0.19	$\chi^2(1) = 120.83$	<0.0001
+ educational level		−0.23 (0.02)	−0.27–0.19	$\chi^2(1) = 134.67$	<0.0001
+ PA × diagnosis groups					
	Persons with current affective disorders				
	Remitted persons †	0.00 (0.05)	−0.09–0.10	$\chi^2(1) = 0.01$	0.92
	Healthy controls †	−0.00 (0.07)	−0.13–0.13	$\chi^2(1) = 0.00$	0.99
+ PA × weekly working hours		0.00 (0.00)	−0.00–0.00	$\chi^2(1) = 0.23$	0.63
+ PA × gender ‡		−0.09 (0.04)	−0.17–0.00	$\chi^2(1) = 3.77$	0.05
+ PA × age		−0.00 (0.00)	−0.00–0.00	$\chi^2(1) = 0.31$	0.58
+ PA × educational level					
	Low				
	Moderate §	−0.07 (0.07)	−0.22–0.08	$\chi^2(1) = 0.90$	0.34
	High §	−0.13 (0.07)	−0.28–0.02	$\chi^2(1) = 3.11$	0.08
Negative affect and momentary burden					
Negative affect (NA) *		0.30 (0.03)	0.24–0.37	$\chi^2(1) = 80.53$	<0.0001
+ diagnosis groups		0.29 (0.03)	0.22–0.36	$\chi^2(1) = 73.09$	<0.0001
+ weekly working hours		0.31 (0.03)	0.24–0.38	$\chi^2(1) = 83.94$	<0.0001
+ gender		0.31 (0.03)	0.24–0.37	$\chi^2(1) = 81.76$	<0.0001
+ age		0.30 (0.03)	0.23–0.37	$\chi^2(1) = 73.79$	<0.0001
+ educational level		0.32 (0.03)	0.25–0.38	$\chi^2(1) = 90.22$	<0.0001
+ NA × diagnosis groups					
	Persons with current affective disorders				
	Remitted persons †	0.05 (0.07)	−0.09–0.19	$\chi^2(1) = 0.48$	0.49
	Healthy controls †	0.09 (0.13)	−0.15–0.40	$\chi^2(1) = 0.54$	0.46
+ NA × weekly working hours		−0.00 (0.00)	−0.01–0.00	$\chi^2(1) = 1.09$	0.30
+ NA × gender ‡		0.04 (0.07)	−0.10–0.18	$\chi^2(1) = 0.33$	0.57
+ NA × age		0.01 (0.00)	−0.00–0.01	$\chi^2(1) = 3.77$	0.05
+ NA × educational level					
	Low				
	Moderate §	0.15 (0.14)	−0.12–0.42	$\chi^2(1) = 1.14$	0.29
	High §	0.21 (0.14)	−0.06–0.49	$\chi^2(1) = 2.28$	0.13
Stability of momentary burden					
Time●		0.00 (0.00)	0.00–0.00	$\chi^2(1) = 2.83$	0.09

Note: Generalized estimated equation models. Models are calculated over the whole sample, with a total of 24,537 completed EMA questionnaires. * Shows the unadjusted models. PA = positive affect, NA = negative affect. If appropriate, covariates diagnosis groups, weekly working hours, gender, age, educational level were separately added to unadjusted models. Hereafter, interaction terms were added to the unadjusted model. For the interaction terms, the regression coefficient of the interaction term is shown. † Persons with current affective disorders used as a reference group, ‡ men are used as reference group, and § low educational level is used as a reference group. ● Stability of momentary burden was measured by adding time to the unadjusted model.

3.2.3. Experienced Burden Over Whole Monitoring Period

We asked the participants to evaluate the overall experienced burden of the whole two-week EMA monitoring period. Figure 3 shows the median (Mdn) and inter-quartile range (IQR) of the overall experienced burden. The persons with current affective disorders reported an average score of 2.5 (n = 95; IQR = 1.50–3.75), the remitted persons 2.25 (n = 182; IQR = 1.25–3.25), and healthy controls 2.0 (n = 92; IQR = 1.00–3.13). No significant inter-group differences regarding average overall experienced burden were found (H[2] = 5.56, p = 0.062).

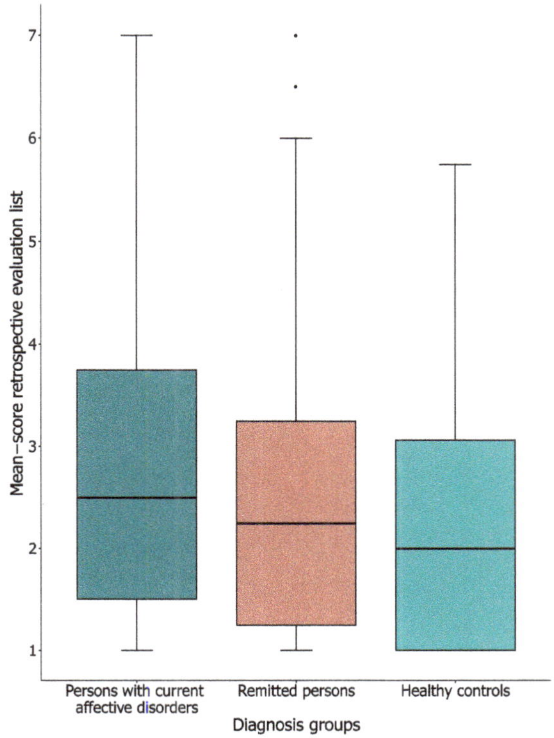

Figure 3. Mean scores of the retrospective evaluation of experienced burden. Note: Mean scores of the retrospective evaluation; a reflection of experienced burden over the whole EMA monitoring period. Score range between 1 and 7, higher score indicates more burden. Thick black line shows the median, error bars show the interquartile range (IQR), whiskers show +/−1.5 IQR, and ● = outlier, deviates by ≥ 1.5× IQR.

3.2.4. Adherence Rates

Adherence to the daily EMA questionnaires was our other main outcome. We looked at adherence rates, self-reported main reasons for missing questionnaires, and the number of omissions due to technical issues. Figure 4 shows the median (Mdn) and inter-quartile range (IQR) of the adherence rates to the EMA questionnaires. All groups showed the same median adherence rate (66 out of 70 [94.3%]) to the EMA measures, meaning that there is no significant difference between the persons with current affective disorders (IQR = 63.5–69.0), the remitted persons (IQR = 63.0–68.0), and the healthy controls (IQR = 62.0–69.0; (H[2] = 0.08, p = 0.98). These results show that adherence rates in our sample were high.

3.2.5. Reasons for Missing Daily EMA Questionnaires

After the last daily EMA questionnaire, participants were asked to list their main reasons for missing questionnaires. In total, 369 participants (out of 384) completed this addendum questionnaire-321 of which missed at least one EMA questionnaire. For 57.2% of them (184 out of 321), it appears that 'being busy with an activity' was one of their main reasons for missing a questionnaire. Other reasons frequently reported were 'no network connection' (reported by 22.4% [72 out of 321]), and 'being asleep' (reported by 21.2% [68 out of 321]). There are no statistically significant group differences for these and the other reasons as listed in Table 3.

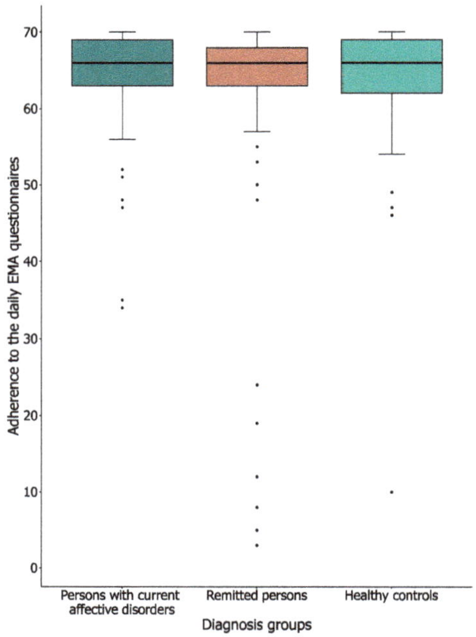

Figure 4. Adherence to the EMA questionnaires. Note: Participants were invited to conduct a total of 70 EMA questionnaires. Thick black line shows the median, error bars show the interquartile range (IQR), whiskers show +/−1.5 IQR, and ● = outlier, deviates by ≥ 1.5× IQR.

Table 3. Self-reported main reasons for missing EMA questionnaires.

	Persons with Current Affective Disorders (n = 77)	Remitted Persons (n = 156)	Healthy Controls (n = 75)	Total (n = 321)	Test Value	p Value
Amount of reasons	2 (1–2)	2 (1–2)	1 (1–2)	2 (1-3)	H(2) = 3.10	0.21
Main reasons for missing questionnaires						
Being busy with an activity	52 (67.5)	86 (55.1)	46 (61.3)	184 (57.3)	$\chi^2(2) = 3.40$	0.18
No network connection	18 (23.4)	38 (24.4)	16 (21.3)	72 (22.4)	$\chi^2(2) = 0.26$	0.88
Being asleep	22 (28.6)	36 (23.1)	10 (13.3)	68 (21.2)	$\chi^2(2) = 5.31$	0.07
Technical problems	14 (18.2)	29 (18.6)	15 (20.0)	58 (18.1)	$\chi^2(2) = 0.94$	0.95
Did not hear the smartphone	17 (22.1)	24 (15.4)	14 (18.7)	55 (17.1)	$\chi^2(2) = 1.62$	0.45
Did not bring the smartphone	12 (15.6)	26 (16.7)	7 (9.3)	45 (14.0)	$\chi^2(2) = 2.26$	0.32
Could not make themselves do it	1 (1.3)	0 (0.0)	0 (0.0)	1 (0.3)	$\chi^2(2) = 3.01$	0.22
Other reason	15 (19.5)	40 (25.6)	18 (24.0)	73 (22.7)	$\chi^2(2) = 1.09$	0.58

Note: Data are n (%) or median (IQR). Only individuals who missed at least one EMA questionnaire and completed the addendum questionnaire were taken into account in this table. Participants were allowed to select more than one option. Likelihood ratio or Pearson's chi-square tests were used as appropriate.

Next, we checked whether EMA questionnaires were missed due to technical issues with the server. In the group of persons with current affective disorders, this was the case for 0.14% (10 out of 7000) of the questionnaires. The equivalent figure for the group of remitted persons was 0.19% (25 out of 13,300) and for the healthy controls it was 0.30% (20 out of 6,580 measures). It thus appears that, across the sample, technical issues accounted for only a small number of the missed questionnaires.

4. Discussion

The results of this study show that, when asked at the moment of assessing, perceived burden as a result of the ecological momentary assessment (EMA) questionnaires was slightly higher when affect was worse. Adhering to the measure was thus more burdensome for persons diagnosed with an affective disorder, than it was for remitted persons and healthy controls. Nevertheless, when asked to evaluate the overall experienced burden of the whole two-week monitoring period, no significant inter-group differences were found. Moreover, the persons with current affective disorders showed very high adherence rates regardless.

Our findings show that when asked "in the moment", higher negative affect and lower positive affect were associated with slightly higher levels of perceived burden as a result of the EMA questionnaires. This was the case for all diagnosis groups and regardless the number of weekly working hours, age, gender, and educational background of the participant. The persons with current affective disorders thus reported higher levels of burden by comparison to the other two groups. These findings could possibly be explained by the fact that the clinical picture of the current affective disorders involves a persistent depressed mood and/or diminished interest or pleasure in general [17,18]. Adhering to EMA questionnaires might therefore be more intrusive to persons with current affective disorders, than for persons without such a disorder. Nevertheless, across the two-week EMA monitoring period the experienced burden remained stable, and for the overall experienced burden of the whole two-week EMA inter-group differences were no longer found.

Importantly, the higher levels of "in the moment burden" amongst the persons with current affective disorders did not result in nonadherence; on average, they completed over 94% of the EMA questionnaires—a rate on a par with the other two groups in this cohort. Moreover, the adherence rates found in this study are even higher than in previous ones with a similar population, although these studies used different EMA methods (e.g., paper-and-pencil diaries, PDAs) [8,14,15]. Previous studies using a smartphone-based method in other psychiatric populations also had lower adherence. A meta-analysis showed a pooled average adherence rate of 71% in substance abusers [30]. Note, however, the adherence rates in our study might have been influenced by the fact that participants were allowed to answer the questionnaires within 60 minutes after being prompted. Other studies often only allow for a short period of time to complete the questionnaires (e.g., up till 30 minutes) [31].

Our study does have some limitations, though, which should be considered when interpreting our findings. Most notably, it can be reasonably assumed that the participants in the NESDA-EMAA sample are highly motivated as they have been taking part in the NESDA study for over nine years. In addition, the results of our a relatively short EMA monitoring period might not be readily generalized to other settings that rely on longer EMA monitoring periods. Another point is that momentary burden was collected with one single item As a result, the psychometric properties of this main outcome measure could not be assessed. In future work, it is advised to include (multiple item) questionnaires in order to report psychometric properties of the momentary burden assessment. Still, the results of the present study have important clinical implications for clinical practice. In most clinical settings, some form of real-time data is already gathered via paper-and-pencil methods (e.g., thought diaries, assessment of mood fluctuation in bipolar patients, or assessments of the frequency and intensity of panic attacks). The number of studies investigating the clinical usefulness of EMA methods via a smartphone in routine practice is also rising [32–34]. User experiences should also be explored in clinical settings when considering whether EMA can indeed be translated into a tool, beneficial for patients with affective disorders.

5. Conclusions

In conclusion, even though the persons with current affective disorders did report experiencing more burden as a result of the EMA questionnaires when asked about this at the moment of assessment, this was not the case when asked to evaluate the whole monitoring period, and they were still able and willing to provide real-time information on their mental well-being. This study is, to the best of our knowledge, the first to systematically examine user experiences of EMA questionnaires in persons with current affective disorders while making a direct comparison with remitted persons and healthy controls in a single cohort. Although our conclusions highlight the need to examine this topic further, they do already provide important insights into the acceptability of (short-duration) EMA methods for persons with affective disorders.

Author Contributions: All authors have contributed substantially to the work reported. All authors critically revised the paper. Conceptualization, C.R.v.G., J.S., H.M.R. and J.H.S.; methodology, C.R.v.G., J.S., H.M.R. and J.H.S.; writing—original draft preparation, C.R.v.G.; writing—review and editing, J.S., F.L., H.R., B.W.J.H.P., R.A.S., H.M.R. and J.H.S.; supervision: J.S., H.M.R. and J.H.S. All authors have read and agreed to the published version of the manuscript.

Acknowledgments: This work was financially supported by Innovative Medicines Initiative 2 Joint undertaking under grant agreement no. 115902. Femke Lamers has received funding from the European Union Seventh Framework Programme (FP7/2007–2013) under grant agreement no. PCIG12-GA-2012-334065. The infrastructure for the NESDA study (www.nesda.nl) is funded through the Geestkracht program of the Netherlands Organization for Health Research and Development (ZonMw, grant number no. 10-000-1002) and financial contributions by participating universities and mental health care organizations (Amsterdam UMC location VUmc, GGZ inGeest, Leiden University Medical Centre, Leiden University, GGZ Rivierduinen, University Medical Centre Groningen, University of Groningen, Lentis, GGZ Friesland, GGZ Drenthe, Rob Giel Onderzoekscentrum).

Conflicts of Interest: B.P has received (non-related) grant funding from Boehringer Ingelheim and Jansen Research. All other authors declare that they have no competing interests.

References

1. Houben, M.; van den Noortgate, W.; Kuppens, P. The Relation between Short-Term Emotion Dynamics and Psychological Well-Being: A Meta-Analysis. *Psychol. Bull.* **2015**, *141*, 901–930. [CrossRef] [PubMed]
2. Lamers, L.; Swendsen, J.; Cui, L.; Husky, M.; Johns, J.; Zipunnikov, V.; Merikangas, K.R. Mood Reactivity and Affective Dynamics in Mood and Anxiety Disorders. *J. Abnorm. Psychol.* **2018**, *127*, 659–669. [CrossRef] [PubMed]
3. Nelson, J.; Klumparendt, A.; Doebler, P.; Ehring, T. Everyday Emotional Dynamics in Major Depression. *Emotion* **2018**. [CrossRef] [PubMed]
4. Thompson, R.J.; Mata, J.; Jaeggi, S.M.; Buschkuehl, M.; Jonides, J.; Gotlib, I.H. The everyday emotional experience of adults with major depressive disorder: Examining emotional instability, inertia, and reactivity. *J. Abnorm. Psychol.* **2012**, *121*, 819–829. [CrossRef] [PubMed]
5. Marzano, L.; Bardill, A.; Fields, B.; Herd, K.; Veale, D.; Grey, N.; Moran, P. The Application of MHealth to Mental Health: Opportunities and Challenges. *Lancet Psychiatry* **2015**, *2*, 942–948. [CrossRef]
6. Myin-Germeys, I.; Kasanova, Z.; Vaessen, T.; Vachon, H.; Kirtley, O.; Viechtbauer, W.; Reininghaus, U. Experience Sampling Methodology in Mental Health Research: New Insights and Technical Developments. *World Psychiatry* **2018**, *17*, 123–132. [CrossRef]
7. Trull, T.J.; Ebner-Priemer, U.W. Using Experience Sampling Methods/Ecological Momentary Assessment (ESM/EMA) in Clinical Assessment and Clinical Research: Introduction to the Special Section. *Psychol. Assess.* **2009**, *21*, 457–462. [CrossRef]
8. Wenze, S.J.; Miller, I.W. Use of Ecological Momentary Assessment in Mood Disorders Research. *Clin. Psychol. Rev.* **2010**, *30*, 794–804. [CrossRef]
9. Shiffman, S.; Stone, A.A.; Hufford, M.R. Ecological Momentary Assessment. *Ann. Rev. Clin. Psychol.* **2008**, *4*, 1–32. [CrossRef]
10. Ben-Zeev, D.; Young, M.A.; Madsen, J.W. Retrospective Recall of Affect in Clinically Depressed Individuals and Controls. *Cogn. Emot.* **2009**, *23*, 1021–1040. [CrossRef]
11. Gloster, A.T.; Miché, M.; Wersebe, H.; Mikoteit, T.; Hoyer, J.; Imboden, C.; Bader, K.; Meyer, A.H.; Hatzinger, M.; Lieb, R. Daily Fluctuation of Emotions and Memories Thereof: Design and Methods of an Experience Sampling Study of Major Depression, Social Phobia, and Controls. *Int. J. Methods Psychiatr. Res.* **2017**, *26*, 1–12. [CrossRef] [PubMed]
12. Myin-Germeys, I.; Oorschot, M.; Collip, D.; Lataster, J.; Delespaul, P.; van Os, J. Experience Sampling Research in Psychopathology: Opening the Black Box of Daily Life. *Psychol. Med.* **2009**, *39*, 1533–1547. [CrossRef] [PubMed]

13. Armey, M.F.; Schatten, H.T.; Haradhvala, N.; Miller, I.W. Ecological momentary assessment (EMA) of depression-related phenomena. *Curr. Opin. Psychol.* **2015**, *4*, 21–25. [CrossRef] [PubMed]
14. Aan het Rot, M.; Hogenelst, K.; Schoevers, R.A. Mood Disorders in Everyday Life A Systematic Review of Experience Sampling and Ecological Momentary Assessment Studies. *Clin. Psychol. Rev.* **2012**, *32*, 510–523. [CrossRef]
15. Colombo, D.; Fernández-Álvarez, J.; Patané, A.; Semonella, M.; Kwiatkowska, M.; García-Palacios, A.; Cipresso, P.; Riva, G.; Botella, C. Current State and Future Directions of Technology-Based Ecological Momentary Assessment and Intervention for Major Depressive Disorder: A Systematic Review. *J. Clin. Med.* **2019**, *8*, 465. [CrossRef]
16. Walz, L.C.; Nauta, M.H.; Aan Het Rot, M. Experience Sampling and Ecological Momentary Assessment for Studying the Daily Lives of Patients with Anxiety Disorders: A Systematic Review. *J. Anxiety Disord.* **2014**, *28*, 925–937. [CrossRef]
17. American Psychiatric Association. *Diagnostic and Statistical Manual of Mental Disorders*, 5th ed.; American Psychiatric Association: Washington, DC, USA, 2013.
18. Beck, A.T.; Alford, B.A. *Depression: Causes and Treatment*, 2nd ed.; University of Pennsylvania Press: Philadelphia, PL, USA, 2009.
19. Difrancesco, S.; Lamers, F.; Riese, H.; Merikangas, K.R.; Beekman, A.T.F.; Hemert, A.M.; Schoevers, R.A.; Penninx, B.W.J.H. Sleep, Circadian Rhythm, and Physical Activity Patterns in Depressive and Anxiety Disorders: A 2-week Ambulatory Assessment Study. *Depress. Anxiety* **2019**. [CrossRef]
20. Schoevers, R.A.; Van Borkulo, C.D.; Lamers, F.; Servaas, M.N.; Bastiaansen, J.A.C.J.; Beekman, A.T.; Van Hemert, A.M.; Smit, J.H.; Penninx, B.W.J.H.; Riese, H. Momentary affect fluctuations differ between patients with current depression and anxiety disorders, remitters and healthy controls. *Psychol. Med.* (under review).
21. Penninx, B.W.J.H.; Beekman, A.T.; Smit, J.H.; Zitman, F.G.; Nolen, W.A.; Spinhoven, P.; Cuijpers, P.; De Jong, P.J.; Van Marwijk, H.W.; Assendelft, W.J.; et al. The Netherlands Study of Depression and Anxiety (NESDA): Rationale, Objectives and Methods. *Int. J. Methods Psychiatr. Res.* **2008**, *17*, 121–140. [CrossRef]
22. Sytema, S.; van der Krieke, L. Routine Outcome Monitoring: A Tool to Improve the Quality of Mental Health Care. In *Improving Mental Health Care: The Global Challenge*, 1st ed.; Thornicroft, G., Ruggeri, M., Goldberg, D., Eds.; John Wiley & Sons: Chichester, UK, 2013.
23. Bouwmans, C.; De Jong, K.; Timman, R.; Zijlstra-Vlasveld, M.; Van Der Feltz-Cornelis, C.; Tan, S.S.; Hakkaart-Van Roijen, L. Feasibility, reliability and validity of a questionnaire on healthcare consumption and productivity loss in patients with a psychiatric disorder (TiC-P). *BMC Health Serv. Res.* **2013**, *13*, 217. [CrossRef]
24. American Psychiatric Association. *Diagnostic and Statistical Manual of Mental Disorders*, 4th ed.; American Psychiatric Association: Washington, DC, USA, 1994.
25. WHO. *Composite International Diagnostic Interview*, version 2.1; World Health Organization: Geneva, Switzerland, 1991.
26. Wittchen, H.U.; Robins, L.N.; Cottler, L.B.; Sartorius, N.; Burke, J.D.; Regier, D. Cross-Cultural Feasibility, Reliability and Sources of Variance of the Composite International Diagnostic Interview (CIDI). *Br. J. Psychiatr.* **1991**, *159*, 645–653. [CrossRef]
27. Bennik, E. Every Dark Cloud Has a Colored Lining: The Relation between Positive and Negative Affect and Reactivity to Positive and Negative Events. Ph.D. Thesis, University of Groningen, Groningen, The Netherlands, 2015.
28. Lu, B.; Preisser, J.S.; Qaqish, B.F.; Suchindran, C.; Bangdiwala, S.I.; Wolfson, M. A comparison of two bias-corrected covariance estimators for generalized estimating equations. *Biometrics* **2007**, *63*, 935–941. [CrossRef] [PubMed]
29. Twisk, J.; de Vente, W. Attrition in Longitudinal Studies: How to Deal with Missing Data. *J. Clin. Epidemiol.* **2002**, *55*, 329–337. [CrossRef]
30. Jones, A.; Remmerswaal, D.; Verveer, I.; Robinson, E.; Franken, I.H.A.; Wen, C.K.F.; Field, M. Compliance with Ecological Momentary Assessment Protocols in Substance Users: A Meta-Analysis. *Addiction* **2018**, *114*, 609–619. [CrossRef] [PubMed]
31. Janssens, K.A.M.; Bos, E.H.; Rosmalen, J.G.M.; Wichers, M.C.; Riese, H. A Qualitative Approach to Guide Choices for Designing a Diary Study. *BMC Med. Res. Methodol.* **2018**, *18*. [CrossRef] [PubMed]

32. Bos, F.M.; Snippe, E.; Bruggeman, R.; Wichers, M.; van der Krieke, L. Insights of patients and clinicians on the promise of the experience sampling method for psychiatric care. *Psychiatr. Serv.* **2019**, *70*, 983–991. [CrossRef]
33. Loo Gee, B.; Griffiths, K.M.; Gulliver, A. Effectiveness of Mobile Technologies Delivering Ecological Momentary Interventions for Stress and Anxiety: A Systematic Review. *J. Am. Med. Inform. Assoc.* **2016**, *23*, 221–229. [CrossRef]
34. Schueller, S.M.; Aguilera, A.; Mohr, D.C. Ecological Momentary Interventions for Depression and Anxiety. *Depress. Anxiety* **2017**. [CrossRef]

Journal of
Clinical Medicine

MDPI

Article

From Research to Practice: Ten Lessons in Delivering Digital Mental Health Services

Nickolai Titov [1,*], Heather D. Hadjistavropoulos [2], Olav Nielssen [1], David C. Mohr [3], Gerhard Andersson [4,5] and Blake F. Dear [1]

1 MindSpot Clinic and Department of Psychology, Macquarie University, Sydney, NSW 2109, Australia
2 Online Therapy Unit, Department of Psychology, University of Regina, Regina, Saskatchewan, SK S4S 0A2, Canada
3 Center for Behavioral Intervention Technologies, Department of Preventive Medicine, Northwestern University, Chicago, IL 60611, USA
4 Department of Behavioural Sciences and Learning, Linköping University, Linköping SE-581 83, Sweden
5 Department of Clinical Neuroscience, Karolinska Institute, Stockholm 171 77, Sweden
* Correspondence: nick.titov@mq.edu.au

Received: 16 July 2019; Accepted: 15 August 2019; Published: 17 August 2019

Abstract: There is a large body of research showing that psychological treatment can be effectively delivered via the internet, and Digital Mental Health Services (DMHS) are now delivering those interventions in routine care. However, not all attempts to translate these research outcomes into routine care have been successful. This paper draws on the experience of successful DMHS in Australia and Canada to describe ten lessons learned while establishing and delivering internet-delivered cognitive behavioural therapy (ICBT) and other mental health services as part of routine care. These lessons include learnings at four levels of analysis, including lessons learned working with (1) consumers, (2) therapists, (3) when operating DMHS, and (4) working within healthcare systems. Key themes include recognising that DMHS should provide not only treatment but also information and assessment services, that DMHS require robust systems for training and supervising therapists, that specialist skills are required to operate DMHS, and that the outcome data from DMHS can inform future mental health policy. We also confirm that operating such clinics is particularly challenging in the evolving funding, policy, and regulatory context, as well as increasing expectations from consumers about DMHS. Notwithstanding the difficulties of delivering DMHS, we conclude that the benefits of such services for the broader community significantly outweigh the challenges.

Keywords: delivery; implementation; internet-delivered cognitive behaviour therapy; psychological treatment; routine care; depression; anxiety disorders

1. Introduction

Globally, mood and anxiety disorders affect more than 700 million people each year and are associated with considerable burden and disability [1,2]. However, in a 12-month period, fewer than half of those affected seek or receive evidence-based treatments [3–5] for reasons that include cost, limited availability of services in many areas, limited awareness of both illness and the potential benefit of treatment, stigma and preference to self-manage [6].

Delivering psychological services via the internet is one way of increasing access to care. A large number of randomised controlled trials have demonstrated that internet-delivered cognitive behavioural therapy (ICBT) is effective at treating anxiety and depression [7–10]. However, attempts to extend ICBT to routine care have produced mixed results. Several attempts at implementation have either been unsuccessful [11] or were not found to have added value to existing face to face services [12], which has raised doubt as to whether internet-delivered psychological services can be implemented successfully in typical health care settings [13]. Notwithstanding the challenges, the successful use of ICBT as part of routine clinical care has been reported in Sweden [14–17], the Netherlands [18,19], Norway, Denmark [20,21], Canada [22–25], and Australia [26–30]. In addition to reports of outcomes from individual clinics, and reflecting the maturing state of the field, there is now an increasing number of studies describing barriers [20,23,31,32], guidelines for implementation [33,34], and comparisons of clinics across different countries [35]. The successful clinics typically deliver ICBT interventions via so-called virtual or digital mental health services (DMHS). Common features of the successful clinics include high standards of both clinical and organisational governance, and robust systems for staff training and supervision [35].

This paper describes key lessons learned during our own efforts to develop and deliver DMHS. The MindSpot Clinic, Australia, and the Online Therapy Unit (OTU) in the province of Saskatchewan, Canada accept referrals directly from consumers as well as via general practitioners. Together, these DMHS have provided assessments to more than 100,000 people and treatment to more than 30,000 people. The authors have worked closely together for several years and have served on advisory bodies to each other's services. The lessons we describe draw on our shared experiences in service development, delivery and collaboration.

We narrowed down our experience to ten key lessons that were not fully described in other papers. These lessons were not immediately apparent to us when we set about translating our research findings to routine care but have been of fundamental importance in how we developed and now operate our DMHS. Hence, we anticipate that these lessons may help those launching similar clinics.

We intentionally avoided specific frameworks of reporting [36,37], because an aim of this paper was to describe the experiences of operating mature services, rather than just the implementation phase. We also acknowledge that some of these lessons overlap, may not apply in other jurisdictions or even to other DMHS within our own countries.

2. Lessons

We chose to organise our lessons according to the model shown in Table 1, which represents the lessons learned from working with (1) consumers, (2) therapists, (3) operating DMHS, and (4) when operating in the broader health systems, including when engaging with funders and policy makers.

Table 1. Lessons learned at four levels of analysis of digital mental health services (DMHS).

Level	Lesson
1. Consumers	1. DMHS can improve access to care for those who really need care 2. DMHS deliver more than treatment services 3. DMHS are used by a broad cross-section of the population
2. Therapists	1. DMHS require specialised therapist skills 2. DMHS require specialised clinical processes
3. Operating DMHS	1. The operation of DMHS require specialised systems and skills 2. DMHS evolve
4. Health Systems, Funders, and Policy Makers	1. Integrating DMHS within health systems is challenging 2. DMHS may change the mental health system 3. DMHS are not a panacea

Before further describing the lessons learned, key aspects of the MindSpot Clinic and OTU are summarised below.

2.1. The MindSpot Clinic, Sydney, Australia

MindSpot was launched in 2013 and operates from Macquarie University, Sydney. MindSpot is funded by the Australian Government Department of Health, with funding initially provided for a 3-year period as a result of the competitive tender process. MindSpot aims to improve access to evidence-based education, triage, assessment, referral, and treatment services throughout Australia to adults with symptoms of depression and anxiety [28,29]. Clinic services are provided free of charge.

Patients can either self-refer after learning about MindSpot via the website (mindspot.org.au), online advertising, links from other mental health websites, recommendations by previous users or can take up referrals from health professionals. Patients first register online or via telephone and complete a detailed assessment questionnaire followed by telephone or secure email contact with a therapist to discuss symptoms and treatment options. Patients then choose between information to assist with self-management, referral to another service or ICBT. The clinic offers seven ICBT programs that have been validated in clinical trials, including transdiagnostic treatments designed to treat symptoms of anxiety and depression in several age groups [24,38–47] and disorder-specific treatments for obsessive compulsive disorder [48,49], post-traumatic stress disorder [50], and chronic pain [51]. All the treatment programs comprise of five lessons which provide the core information, delivered over eight-weeks. Additional resources targeting specific symptoms or difficulties are made available during treatment to assist patients tailor treatment to their own needs. Outcomes are measured using validated symptom scales that are administered weekly during treatment, on completion, and at a three-month follow-up. The therapists are all registered or provisionally registered mental health professionals who contact and monitor participants weekly during treatment via a secure email system or by telephone. The treatment patients are enrolled in cohorts every two weeks, with therapists each responsible for 50 or so patients. To date, more than 100,000 people have registered to use the clinic, and 25,000 have opted to receive ICBT.

2.2. Online Therapy Unit, Canada

The OTU has operated from the University of Regina in Saskatchewan since October 2010. Initial funding was provided by a federal research grant, but since 2015, the OTU has received stable funding from the Saskatchewan Ministry of Health. The OTU aims to provide therapist-guided ICBT for depression and anxiety and to educate providers of mental health care and conduct research on ICBT in routine practice [25]. Clinic services are also provided to patients free of charge.

The OTU promotes services to patients via word of mouth primarily from health care providers, media reports, and both digital and print communication. Patients are encouraged to visit the clinic online (onlinetherapyuser.ca) and can either self-refer or are referred by a health professional. Patients first complete an online screening followed by telephone assessment.

The OTU delivers several ICBT programs including an adaptation of the Wellbeing course developed at Macquarie University and used at the MindSpot Clinic [44,47,52]. Clinically validated patient reported outcome measures (PROMS) of anxiety and depression are administered regularly during treatment, at post-treatment, and at three-month follow-up. Therapists are registered mental health professionals or graduate students under supervision employed by the clinic or by publicly funded community clinics located in other parts of Saskatchewan. During treatment, patients receive weekly therapist contact primarily via secure email or by telephone to assist in applying the skills taught during treatment. Since October 2010, the clinic had assessed more than 5400 patients, 4200 of whom have received ICBT [23,24,35].

3. The Ten Lessons

3.1. Level 1: Lessons Working with Consumers

The first three lessons refer to the way DMHS can improve access to care and serve a broad section of the community, and how they deliver services other than treatment.

3.1.1. Lesson 1: DMHS Can Improve Access to Care for Those Who Really Need Care

One of the most profound lessons we learned is that DMHS improve access to mental health services for many people who would not otherwise seek care. For example, at least a third of the users of both MindSpot and OTU report that they have not previously spoken to a health professional about symptoms and 80% of MindSpot and 55% of OTU users are not using other mental health services at the time of assessment [28,53].

The users of these services often have chronic and disabling symptoms. A third of MindSpot users have been troubled by their symptoms for between one and five years with a further third reporting symptoms for more than six years. Among users of the OTU, 45% report symptoms for two or more years and those in paid employment report an average of 7 days off work in the last 30 days due to symptoms. Moreover, the mean symptom scores reported by users of MindSpot are in the moderate–severe range, a quarter report suicidal thoughts and 2.4% disclose suicidal plans.

We were also surprised at how people use our DMHS. While most users access content online, many others download information and refer to it when they do not have internet access [54]. In addition, for those who prefer or require printed materials, we send all the treatment course content in printed form [28]. For these reasons, we sometimes think of our services as delivering *virtual* rather than *digital* care, however, we are reluctant to introduce new terms to describe this already definitionally challenged field.

3.1.2. Lesson 2: DMHS Deliver More than Treatment

Contrary to our expectations, not all consumers using our DMHS seek treatment, especially in Australia, where most users report they are primarily seeking a confidential assessment and recommendations about treatment options. This should not have come as a complete surprise, given the high proportion who had not previously sought treatment. However, we learned that for many people, the assessment itself serves as a brief but helpful clinical intervention, particularly when the consumer and therapist create a shared clinical formulation, discuss treatment options that include self-help strategies, and explore barriers and facilitators to recovery. This assessment process is highly regarded by the patients of both clinics.

Consumers also frequently report enormous difficulty understanding and navigating the existing mental health service eco-system and some report using our services to seek advice about other health services, a theme which we return to below. Consequently, our second lesson is that DMHS need to offer a range of services in addition to online treatment, including information, assessment, triage and referral to other services. It should be noted that there are differences between our two clinics, with more people using the OTU reporting they are seeking treatment compared with users of MindSpot [55]. Thus, the specific services offered by DMHS may vary between jurisdictions, possibly reflecting differences in how the clinics are perceived and promoted, and differences in the needs of the local community.

3.1.3. Lesson 3: DMHS are used by a Broad Cross Section of the Population

Our third lesson is that a diverse cross section of our communities access our services, including indigenous Australians and Canadians [56], people on low incomes, people living in rural and remote regions, and other groups who often under-utilise traditional health services. We stress that our DMHS are not a panacea in this regard. Instead, we note that the widespread use of internet-enabled devices to access a range of services, including education, banking, entertainment and other domains, has extended to healthcare. In a similar way, DMHS have considerable potential to reduce, to some degree, the inequality of access to mental health.

A striking example is the ability of DMHS to reach people living in rural areas. Almost 40% of MindSpot users report living outside major metropolitan areas, with many living in rural or remote parts of Australia, including islands off the mainland. Similarly, 28% of OTU users are from rural locations and 32% from small cities. Collectively, these people live in locations where access to health services is limited or sometimes non-existent [55]. A further example relates to engagement by older adults. Across both clinics, approximately 6% of users are over the age of 60, which is a group that often experience difficulty accessing mental health services, including for reasons related to physical impairments. The experience at both clinics is that older adults strongly engage in treatments and often obtain large improvements in symptoms [42].

A final example relates to socio-economic disadvantage. A recent analysis of MindSpot data found that users come from all socio-economic backgrounds, including 33% from the lower four deciles of socio-economic status, a group who are more prone to experience a disadvantage and difficulties accessing mental health services.

3.2. Level 2: Lessons Working with Therapists

Both clinics have now trained large numbers of therapists, previously experienced in delivering face-to-face care, to deliver DMHS. Key lessons have been that therapists working in DMHS require specialised skills and therefore, require specialised training and supervision to acquire and maintain those skills.

3.2.1. Lesson 4: DMHS Require Specialised Therapist Skills

An important lesson is that the skills and knowledge required for effective delivery of DMHS are sufficiently different to those associated with traditional models of care to warrant specialised training and supervision [57]. Obvious examples include the need for DMHS therapists to become competent in the use of clinical software platforms and in engaging with patients via telephone or text-based communication, including responding appropriately to very long messages or technical questions, skills that are not taught in most clinical training programs [23,40,58].

However, there are less obvious reasons for providing specialised training and supervision. First, therapists new to DMHS often intellectually understand that DMHS treatments can result in similar outcomes to face-to-face treatment [10,59] but may initially expect DMHS treatments to produce poorer outcomes, a sentiment they may communicate to consumers [23]. New therapists also often find that their assumptions about mechanisms or facilitators of recovery are challenged, particularly when they learn that DMHS patients can develop very strong therapeutic alliances [60] and may obtain large clinical improvements, even after choosing not to have regular therapist contact [55]. Related to this, therapists are often surprised to learn that the structured educational aspects and resources associated with DMHS offer significant advantages over traditional clinical care where such resources may not be used.

A second reason for providing specialised training and supervision is to support DMHS therapists to successfully process the transference and other dynamics that occur when delivering DMHS to large groups of patients at once. An example of this is the temporary increase in symptoms experienced by many consumers at mid-treatment when they begin to apply skills learned in treatment in their everyday lives. These lapses usually resolve and most continue to recover. This process is familiar to experienced therapists, who can help patients understand this trajectory and can manage their own reactions. However, the effect can be magnified by the large numbers of patients in each treatment cohort, leading to feelings of intense elation or sometimes disillusionment, particularly when some patients choose not to engage with the therapist but have not made this clear at the outset. A strong framework of training and supervision can assist therapists to understand and adapt to these patterns and maintain confidence in both their own performance and the effectiveness of the treatment programs.

3.2.2. Lesson 5: DMHS Require Specialised Clinical Processes

This lesson reflects important differences in the clinical procedures and processes used in DMHS compared to traditional mental health clinics. An obvious example is the use of structured ICBT interventions, questionnaires and outcome measures used in DMHS, the delivery of which are governed by procedures which regulate therapists' actions more than they would in typical in face-to-face services.

This level of structure reflects how DMHS attempt to manage both quality assurance and treatment to large numbers of consumers. Therapists experienced in working at DMHS can efficiently deliver individualised care within these structured frameworks, but this is more difficult for less experienced therapists. Another lesson has been the importance of robust systems for not only training and supervision [58,61], but also the recruitment and retention of clinicians who are comfortable with relatively high levels of structure and process [23].

Another example of how DMHS differ from traditional face-to-face mental health services, at least in our jurisdictions, relates to the use of PROMS and patient-reported experience measures (PREMS) [62–64]. Despite the documented utility of PROMS and PREMS in clinical care, they are infrequently used in traditional services, and rarely as a therapeutic tool for guiding discussions or decisions about treatment or as a method for improving the quality of care. Since our clinics routinely administer PROMS and PREMS during and after treatment, we provide specific training for new therapists to increase their comfort and competence in using measures of outcome and experience [61].

3.3. *Level 3: Lessons Operating Services*

3.3.1. Lesson 6: The Operation of DMHS Require Specialised Systems and Skills

This lesson is obvious, but we include it here because we underestimated the complexity of developing and delivering safe and effective DMHS. We expected that our DMHS would be similar to traditional face-to-face clinical mental health services or an extension of the operations used in our large-scale clinical research trials. However, we quickly learned that safely and effectively operating DMHS required attention in at least four areas.

First, DMHS require robust procedures to define and effectively manage safety risks for people presenting with more severe and complex needs than seen in our clinical trials [30] and who often live in remote locations. This requires developing expertise in evaluation of risk via telephone or online communication, the ability to contact emergency services that are available near where the patient is located, how to refer to such services, and how to stay abreast of changes in their referral and contact details.

Second, although operating DMHS involve similar skills as those required for operating traditional mental health services, including management, human resources, marketing and IT [25], we found that DMHS were sufficiently different to warrant employing people with additional expertise, including skills relevant to telehealth, social media and online marketing.

Third, and in addition to the urgent requirement for establishing robust systems of organizational and clinical governance we recognised that in order to effectively lead our services, we personally needed to develop commercial and management skills, domains in which we, as clinical researchers, had little or no experience. We also needed to address challenges relating to regulation; for example at MindSpot, we needed to determine which of the myriad of possible regulatory frameworks applied to our activities [65] given that most [66] had been developed for traditional face-to-face services. Within the OTU, a similar issue requiring attention was how to meet the different regulatory requirements for services provided by therapists from psychology and social work.

Establishing, maintaining, and subsequently improving our operational systems has required a considerable work effort. Whilst we have recruited specialist staff to assist with such efforts, due to the novelty of DMHS, we often also sometimes found it necessary to train and develop our own staff in these operational and managerial roles.

3.3.2. Lesson 7: Digital Mental Health Clinics Evolve

This lesson represents another difference between DMHS and traditional clinical services. Traditional services may change frequently, but the change is usually limited to organisational structure or branding, with less frequent changes to the service or delivery models. By contrast, our DMHS regularly undergo significant changes in procedures, systems, and even service delivery models due to developments in research, technology, the changing expectations of consumers, and changes in the policy priorities of the funding bodies. However, the most frequent changes stem from reviewing our outcomes and procedures.

For example, within the OTU, changes within recent years include (1) replacing disorder-specific ICBT programs with a transdiagnostic treatment program in light of the extensive comorbidity found among patients seeking services and the efficiency of delivery compared to disorder-specific programs [24], (2) ongoing trials to determine the best level of support and specialisation by therapists [40,67], and (3) the expansion of services to address other needs in the community, such as ICBT for pain [22].

Regular change has significant implications for the operation of our clinics. For example, management needs systems for reliably collecting and analysing data, the ability to develop and test alternative models, and the skills and authority to make decisions. The individuals given the task of implementing change need project leadership and change management skills and procedures to plan and deploy changes. Furthermore, therapists and other staff need to be prepared for and willing to implement changes. This means that all staff members need to be adaptable and change needs to become part of the culture of the DMHS.

3.4. *Level 4: Lessons Working with Health Systems, Funders, and Policy Makers*

This final group of lessons summarises key learnings derived from working with and influencing health systems, in particular, the future role and value of DMHS within health systems.

3.4.1. Lesson 8: Integrating DMHS within Health Systems Is Challenging

Our DMHS reside within enormously complex health systems which might be more accurately described as interconnected nodes of care rather than true *systems*. For example, mental health services, while all purporting to share the aim of improving mental wellbeing, often target different groups and may be accountable to different policy and regulatory frameworks. Health services also differ with respect to funding, and in both Canada and Australia, funding for different types of mental health services can be provided by the federal government, state/provincial government, state mental health commissions, non-governmental organisations and individual consumers. As a result, mental health services are often fragmented, poorly connected, and difficult for consumers to navigate.

The complexity of health systems and their resistance to change created a number of threats to the sustainability and stability of our DMHS, particularly in our early years of service delivery. We were able to overcome such challenges by building strong relationships with key stakeholders and in particular, by publishing outcome data that documented the value of the services. This data has also assisted in defining the role of DMHS in the broader mental healthcare system, including as services which improve access to patients who would otherwise not access mental health services.

These so-called external-facing activities have required considerable time and effort. Participation in such activities has required us to learn the sometimes-subtle rules of engaging with other organisations, to commit to regular participation in networking activities, and to make frequent efforts to build and maintain collaborations. Such activities can be enormously time consuming but we have found that they are an essential component of successfully delivering our DMHS.

3.4.2. Lesson 9: DMHS May Change the Mental Health System

By providing services to large numbers of consumers and because of our routine collection of outcome data, our clinics are having a growing influence on the health system and are increasingly seen as agents or examples of change. In Canada, the experiences and activities of the OTU have influenced the development of e-mental health in several ways [68]. In Australia, data from MindSpot has helped inform long-term government planning and funding strategies for mental health services [69], not only DMHS. The data and outcome driven reports prepared by our services are often in marked contrast to submissions by other groups, which may be based more on opinion rather than on evidence. Hence, an important role of DMHS is to inform policy makers and funders to help improve the broader mental health system by presenting data drawn from a broad cross section of the community and also to nudge traditional services to adopt systems of measurement and reporting of outcomes.

3.4.3. Lesson 10: DMHS Are Not a Panacea

We are struck by how often mental health funders and policy makers, when presented with the evidence from our DMHS, become enthusiastic about their potential without an appreciation of their limits. These limits include the so-called digital divide, that is, the group in society who does not use digital devices, those with very low levels of literacy, and those in crisis, who can benefit from contact with DMHS, but may be better off with a mental health service that includes direct human interaction, as well as those who prefer to see someone face-to-face.

In all our communication, we emphasise that DMHS should complement and not replace existing services. We also emphasise that attention must be paid to systematically evaluating delivery methods that combine the best elements of DMHS with traditional services, including blended care [70–74]. We also stress that consumer knowledge of DMHS is still limited and that even brief education about DMHS can improve consumer perceptions and uptake of services [75]. These observations lead to our final lesson that whilst acknowledging that DMHS can significantly improve access to safe, clinical and cost-effective care, our DMHS are not a panacea.

4. General Discussion

This paper aimed to assist other emerging DMHS by sharing ten lessons we learned from successfully delivering DMHS to very large numbers of consumers. Some of these lessons might seem obvious, but their importance was not always apparent when we started our services. Several key themes are discussed below, followed by recommendations.

One theme is that we expect that demand for this service model will grow. The number of patients treated using ICBT in the OTU has more than doubled in the past four years. The threshold for accessing this model of care is significantly lower than traditional face-to-face services and consumers are becoming increasingly comfortable with using technology to access a broad range of services, including health services. Along with a growth in numbers, we expect that existing DMHS will become more tailored to different populations, for example, people in certain occupations, different cultures, or who have been referred from different pathways, although our experience is that the extent to which the treatment course materials need to be customised is considerably less than expected [56,76–78].

A second theme is that the workforce requires specialised training, clinical supervision and support. This raises broader issues about workforce planning and training programs. We note that many professional bodies have recognised the importance of education and training of mental health professionals and standards in this model of care [79–82] but that few training programs in any mental health discipline offer courses or training opportunities specifically for digital mental health. The absence of such training opportunities poses significant risks for the future sustainability and quality of the field.

A third theme is that the delivery of DMHS requires specialist skills in both clinical and operational domains. We also note that although the costs to entry of developing a DMHS, especially a low volume service, might be relatively low, the costs of maintaining quality services can be high. Inadequate funding and inadequate organisational governance can affect the reputation, credibility, and therefore, the potential of the emerging field of DMHS [83]. Hence, we strongly encourage anyone seeking to launch a DMHS to carefully consider the governance frameworks that will ensure the safe and sustainable delivery of services, or to consider licensing their interventions to groups who have proven success in implementing similar services.

Another theme is that the field of DMHS is rapidly evolving. We encourage those seeking to start a DMHS to consider trialing different models of care to those currently used by existing DMHS, including testing different levels of therapist support [24,40,55] and testing care which combines both face-to-face and online delivery. We note the important work conducted by our European colleagues on blended care [70–74] and by others on mobile services [13] and encourage collaboration in order to collectively develop the most effective models of care.

Our final theme relates to recognising the true value proposition of DMHS. We maintain that they are not a panacea but instead serve several valuable functions, including as a useful complement to existing services, as a way of improving equity of access to mental health care for common psychological disorders, and as a stepping stone to other services. Over-promising may increase the likelihood of short-term funding, but poorly designed and delivered services might harm consumers, disappoint stakeholders and risk the future of DMHS.

4.1. Recommendations

These observations lead to several recommendations which we encourage those contemplating developing DMHS to consider. First, we recommend that new DMHS recruit not only appropriately skilled therapists, but also people with commercial and professional skills, ideally with experience in digital service delivery. Second, given the unique challenges of DMHS, we recommend the development of both thorough initial training of therapists, as well as of systems for ongoing training and supervision. Third, given the likelihood that demand for DMHS will grow, we strongly encourage that organisations involved in training and certification of mental health professionals add content and training opportunities relevant to the competencies required in DMHS.

Fourth, we recommend that emerging DMHS measure and publish their outcomes, including disappointing and negative effects outcomes [84]. We also encourage DMHS to engage with policy makers and funders to develop mental health policy grounded in evidence rather than in opinion. Finally, we strongly encourage DMHS to engage with their consumers in appropriate co-design and evaluation activities to ensure services are not only effective but acceptable to consumers.

4.2. Strengths and Limitations

We believe that the main strength of this paper stems from the authors' shared experience in launching and steadily improving successful high volume DMHS. However, we acknowledge several weaknesses, including that the list of lessons is non-exhaustive and did not include some of the significant challenges associated with managing funding insecurity or bureaucratic and professional challenges within the field of mental health, topics we will return to in a subsequent publication. We also acknowledge that our experiences may not reflect those of other DMHS.

4.3. Conclusions

This paper described ten key lessons learned by the authors when developing, delivering, and evaluating DMHS. Despite the challenges, provided they are delivered safely, effectively and with strong clinical, operational and organisational governance, we remain highly optimistic about the potential of DMHS to reduce the global burden of the high prevalence of mental disorders.

Author Contributions: Conceptualisation, N.T. and B.F.D.; Writing—Original Draft Preparation, N.T., H.D.H., O.N., and B.F.D.; Writing—Review & Editing, N.T., H.D.H., O.N., D.C.M., G.A. and B.F.D.

Acknowledgments: The Online Therapy Unit is funded by Saskatchewan Ministry of Health. Research conducted by the Unit is currently funded by the Canadian Institutes of Health Research (152917), the Saskatchewan Health Research Foundation, and the Saskatchewan Centre for Patient-Oriented Research. The MindSpot Clinic is funded by the Australian Department of Health and supported by MQ Health, Macquarie University. The authors gratefully acknowledge their funders, supporting institutions, the patients for allowing the use of their data, and their clinical, management, and technical teams for their efforts in launching and operating the Clinics. We also acknowledge the achievements and leadership shown by early and current researchers in the field of psychological internet interventions. Their work has strongly influenced the models and outcomes reported here and continue to inspire our attempts at reducing barriers to evidence-based psychological services.

Conflicts of Interest: H.D.H. is funded by Saskatchewan Ministry of Health to operate the Online Therapy Unit. Research conducted by the Unit is currently funded by the Canadian Institutes of Health Research (152917), the Saskatchewan Health Research Foundation, and the Saskatchewan Centre for Patient-Oriented Research. Funders had no involvement in the design of the paper, collection, analysis, or interpretation of the data. N.T. and B.F.D. are funded by the Australian Government to operate the national MindSpot Clinic. O.N. is a member of a Lundbeck advisory board for an antipsychotic medication. The other authors report no financial relationships with commercial interests. This paper was investigator initiated. It was funded by Departmental funds from the authors' university, which had no role in the design, execution, interpretation, or writing of the study.

References

1. Kessler, R.C.; Aguilar-Gaxiola, S.; Alonso, J.; Chatterji, S.; Lee, S.; Ormel, J.; Üstün, T.B.; Wang, P.S. The global burden of mental disorders: An update from the WHO World Mental Health (WMH) surveys. *Epidemiol. E Psichiatr. Soc.* **2009**, *18*, 23–33. [CrossRef]
2. Whiteford, H.A.; Degenhardt, L.; Rehm, J.; Baxter, A.J.; Ferrari, A.J.; Erskine, H.E.; Charlson, F.J.; Norman, R.E.; Flaxman, A.D.; Johns, N.; et al. Global burden of disease attributable to mental and substance use disorders: Findings from the Global Burden of Disease Study 2010. *Lancet* **2013**, *382*, 1575–1586. [CrossRef]
3. Urbanoski, K.; Inglis, D.; Veldhuizen, S. Service Use and Unmet Needs for Substance Use and Mental Disorders in Canada. *Can J. Psychiat.* **2017**, *62*, 551–559. [CrossRef] [PubMed]
4. Wang, P.S.; Matthias, A.; Borges, G.; Bruffaerts, R.; Chiu, T.; De Girolamo, W.; Fayyad, G.; John, G.; Ronald, C.; Kovess, V.; et al. Steven Delay and failure in treatment seeking after first onset of mental disorders in the World Health Organization's World Mental Health Survey Initiative. *World Psychiatry.* **2007**, *6*, 177–185. [PubMed]
5. Whiteford, H.A.; Buckingham, W.J.; Harris, M.G.; Burgess, P.M.; Pirkis, J.E.; Barendregt, J.J.; Hall, W.D. Estimating treatment rates for mental disorders in Australia. *Aust. Health Rev.* **2014**, *38*, 80–85. [CrossRef] [PubMed]
6. Mojtabai, R.; Olfson, M.; Sampson, N.A.; Jin, R.; Druss, B.; Wang, P.S.; Wells, K.B.; Pincus, H.A.; Kessler, R.C. Barriers to mental health treatment: Results from the National Comorbidity Survey Replication. *Psychol. Med.* **2011**, *41*, 1751–1761. [CrossRef] [PubMed]
7. Andrews, G.; Cuijpers, P.; Craske, M.G.; McEvoy, P.; Titov, N. Computer therapy for the anxiety and depressive disorders is effective, acceptable and practical health care: A meta-analysis. *PLoS ONE* **2010**, *5*, e13196. [CrossRef]
8. Andersson, G.; Titov, N. Advantages and limitations of Internet-based interventions for common mental disorders. *World Psychiatry Off. J. World Psychiatr. Assoc.* **2014**, *13*, 4–11. [CrossRef]
9. Andersson, G.; Carlbring, P.; Titov, N.; Lindefors, N. Internet Interventions for Adults with Anxiety and Mood Disorders: A Narrative Umbrella Review of Recent Meta-Analyses. *Can. J. Psychiatry* **2019**, *64*, 465–470. [CrossRef]
10. Carlbring, P.; Andersson, G.; Cuijpers, P.; Riper, H.; Hedman-Lagerlöf, E. Internet-based vs. face-to-face cognitive behavior therapy for psychiatric and somatic disorders: An updated systematic review and meta-analysis. *Cogn. Behav. Ther.* **2018**, *47*, 1–18. [CrossRef]
11. Gilbody, S.; Littlewood, E.; Hewitt, C.; Brierley, G.; Tharmanathan, P.; Araya, R.; Barkham, M.; Bower, P.; Cooper, C.; Gask, L.; et al. Computerised cognitive behaviour therapy (cCBT) as treatment for depression in primary care (REEACT trial): Large scale pragmatic randomised controlled trial. *BMJ* **2015**. [CrossRef]
12. Kenter, R.M.F.; Van De Ven, P.M.; Cuijpers, P.; Koole, G.; Niamat, S.; Gerrits, R.S.; Willems, M.; Van Straten, A. Costs and effects of Internet cognitive behavioral treatment blended with face-to-face treatment: Results from a naturalistic study. *Internet Interv.* **2015**, *2*, 77–83. [CrossRef]

13. Mohr, D.C.; Weingardt, K.R.; Reddy, M.; Schueller, S.M. Three Problems with Current Digital Mental Health Research and Three Things We Can Do About Them. *Psychiatr. Serv.* **2017**, *68*, 427–429. [CrossRef]
14. El Alaoui, S.; Hedman, E.; Kaldo, V.; Hesser, H.; Kraepelien, M.; Andersson, E.; Rück, C.; Andersson, G.; Ljótsson, B.; Lindefors, N. Effectiveness of Internet-based cognitive–behavior therapy for social anxiety disorder in clinical psychiatry. *J. Consult. Clin. Psychol.* **2015**, *83*, 902. [CrossRef]
15. Hedman, E.; Ljótsson, B.; Kaldo, V.; Hesser, H.; El Alaoui, S.; Kraepelien, M.; Andersson, E.; Rück, C.; Svanborg, C.; Andersson, G.; et al. Effectiveness of Internet-based cognitive behaviour therapy for depression in routine psychiatric care. *J. Affect. Disord.* **2014**, *155*, 49–58. [CrossRef]
16. Hedman, E.; Ljótsson, B.; Rück, C.; Bergström, J.; Andersson, G.; Kaldo, V.; Jansson, L.; Andersson, E.; Andersson, E.; Blom, K.; et al. Effectiveness of Internet-based cognitive behaviour therapy for panic disorder in routine psychiatric care. *Acta Psychiatri. Scand.* **2013**, *128*, 457–467. [CrossRef]
17. Hedman, E.; Ljótsson, B.; Andersson, E.; Rück, C.; Andersson, G.; Lindefors, N. Effectiveness and cost offset analysis of group CBT for hypochondriasis delivered in a psychiatric setting: An open trial. *Cogn. Behav. Ther.* **2010**, *39*, 239–250. [CrossRef]
18. Ruwaard, J.; Lange, A.; Schrieken, B.; Dolan, C.V.; Emmelkamp, P. The Effectiveness of Online Cognitive Behavioral Treatment in Routine Clinical Practice. *Plos One* **2012**, *7*, e40089. [CrossRef]
19. Ruwaard, J.; Lange, A.; Schrieken, B.; Emmelkamp, P.M. Efficacy and effectiveness of online cognitive behavioral treatment: A decade of interapy research. *Stud. Health Technol. Inform.* **2011**, *167*, 9–14.
20. Folker, A.P.; Mathiasen, K.; Lauridsen, S.M.; Stenderup, E.; Dozeman, E.; Folker, M.P. Implementing internet-delivered cognitive behavior therapy for common mental health disorders: A comparative case study of implementation challenges perceived by therapists and managers in five European internet services. *Internet Interv.* **2018**, *11*, 60–70. [CrossRef]
21. Mathiasen, K.; Riper, H.; Ehlers, L.H.; Valentin, J.B.; Rosenberg, N.K. Internet-based CBT for social phobia and panic disorder in a specialised anxiety clinic in routine care: Results of a pilot randomised controlled trial. *Internet Interv.* **2016**, *4*, 92–98. [CrossRef]
22. Hadjistavropoulos, H.D.; Schneider, L.H.; Hadjistavropoulos, T.; Titov, N.; Dear, B.F. Effectiveness, acceptability and feasibility of an Internet-delivered cognitive behavioral pain management program in a routine online therapy clinic in Canada. *Can. J. Pain* **2018**, *2*, 62–73. [CrossRef]
23. Hadjistavropoulos, H.; Nugent, M.; Dirkse, D.; Pugh, N. Implementation of internet-delivered cognitive behavior therapy within community mental health clinics: A process evaluation using the consolidated framework for implementation research. *BMC Psychiatry* **2017**, *17*, 331. [CrossRef]
24. Hadjistavropoulos, H.; Nugent, M.; Alberts, N.; Staples, L.; Dear, B.; Titov, N. Transdiagnostic Internet-delivered cognitive behaviour therapy in Canada: An open trial comparing results of a specialized online clinic and nonspecialized community clinics. *J. Anxiety Disord.* **2016**, *42*, 19–29. [CrossRef]
25. Hadjistavropoulos, H.D.; Thompson, M.; Ivanov, M.; Drost, C.; Butz, C.J.; Klein, B.; Austin, D.W. Considerations in the Development of a Therapist-Assisted Internet Cognitive Behavior Therapy Service. *Prof. Psycol. Res. Pr.* **2011**, *42*, 463–471. [CrossRef]
26. Newby, J.M.; Mackenzie, A.; Williams, A.D.; McIntyre, K.; Watts, S.; Wong, N.; Andrews, G. Internet cognitive behavioural therapy for mixed anxiety and depression: A randomized controlled trial and evidence of effectiveness in primary care. *Psychol. Med.* **2013**, *43*, 2635–2648. [CrossRef]
27. Williams, A.D.; Andrews, G. The Effectiveness of Internet Cognitive Behavioural Therapy (iCBT) for Depression in Primary Care: A Quality Assurance Study. *PloS One* **2013**, *8*, e57447. [CrossRef]
28. Titov, N.; Dear, B.F.; Staples, L.G.; Bennett-Levy, J.; Klein, B.; Rapee, R.M.; Andersson, G.; Purtell, C.; Bezuidenhout, G.; Nielssen, O.B. The first 30 months of the MindSpot Clinic: Evaluation of a national e-mental health service against project objectives. *Aust. New Zealand J. Psychiatry* **2017**, *51*, 1227–1239. [CrossRef]
29. Titov, N.; Dear, B.F.; Staples, L.G.; Bennett-Levy, J.; Klein, B.; Rapee, R.M.; Shann, C.; Richards, D.; Andersson, G.; Ritterband, L.; et al. MindSpot Clinic: An Accessible, Efficient, and Effective Online Treatment Service for Anxiety and Depression. *Psychiatr. Serv.* **2015**, *66*, 1043–1050. [CrossRef]
30. Nielssen, O.; Dear, B.F.; Staples, L.G.; Dear, R.; Ryan, K.; Purtell, C.; Titov, N. Procedures for risk management and a review of crisis referrals from the MindSpot Clinic, a national service for the remote assessment and treatment of anxiety and depression. *BMC Psychiatry* **2015**, *15*, 304. [CrossRef]

31. Mathiasen, K.; Riper, H.; Andersen, T.E.; Roessler, K.K. Evaluation of Clinical Effect in Routine Secondary Care of Guided Internet Based CBT for Adult Depression and Anxiety: An Observational Study. *JMIR Preprints*. **2018**. [CrossRef]
32. Vis, C.; Mol, M.; Kleiboer, A.; Bührmann, L.; Finch, T.; Smit, J.; Riper, H. Improving Implementation of eMental Health for Mood Disorders in Routine Practice: Systematic Review of Barriers and Facilitating Factors. *JMIR Ment. Health* **2018**, *5*, e20. [CrossRef]
33. Vis, C.; Ruwaard, J.; Finch, T.; Rapley, T.; de Beurs, D.; van Stel, H.; van Lettow, B.; Mol, M.; Kleiboer, A.; Riper, H.; et al. Toward an Objective Assessment of Implementation Processes for Innovations in Health Care: Psychometric Evaluation of the Normalization Measure Development (NoMAD) Questionnaire Among Mental Health Care Professionals. *J. Med. Int. Res.* **2019**, *21*, e12376. [CrossRef]
34. ImpleMentAll: Getting eHealth implementation right. Available online: https://www.implementall.eu/ (accessed on 25 June 2019).
35. Titov, N.; Dear, B.; Nielssen, O.; Staples, L.; Hadjistavropoulos, H.; Nugent, M.; Adlam, K.; Nordgreen, T.; Bruvik, K.H.; Hovland, A.; et al. ICBT in routine care: A descriptive analysis of successful clinics in five countries. *Internet Interv.* **2018**, *13*, 108–115. [CrossRef]
36. Damschroder, L.J.; Aron, D.C.; Keith, R.E.; Kirsh, S.R.; Alexander, J.A.; Lowery, J.C. Fostering implementation of health services research findings into practice: A consolidated framework for advancing implementation science. *Implement. Sci.* **2009**, *4*, 50. [CrossRef]
37. Gaglio, B.; Shoup, J.A.; Glasgow, R.E. The RE-AIM framework: A systematic review of use over time. *Am. J. Public Health* **2013**, *103*, e38–e46. [CrossRef]
38. Staples, L.G.; Dear, B.F.; Johnson, B.; Fogliati, V.; Gandy, M.; Fogliati, R.; Nielssen, O.; Titov, N. Internet-delivered treatment for young adults with anxiety and depression: Evaluation in routine clinical care and comparison with research trial outcomes. *J. Affect. Disord.* **2019**, *256*, 103–109. [CrossRef]
39. Dear, B.F.; Fogliati, V.J.; Fogliati, R.; Johnson, B.; Boyle, O.; Karin, E.; Gandy, M.; Kayrouz, R.; Staples, L.G.; Titov, N. Treating anxiety and depression in young adults: A randomised controlled trial comparing clinician-guided versus self-guided Internet-delivered cognitive behavioural therapy. *Aust. New Zealand J. Psychiatry* **2018**, *52*, 668–679. [CrossRef]
40. Hadjistavropoulos, H.D.; Schneider, L.H.; Edmonds, M.; Karin, E.; Nugent, M.N.; Dirkse, D.; Dear, B.F.; Titov, N. Randomized controlled trial of internet-delivered cognitive behaviour therapy comparing standard weekly versus optional weekly therapist support. *J. Anxiety Disord.* **2017**, *52*, 15–24. [CrossRef]
41. Fogliati, V.J.; Dear, B.F.; Staples, L.G.; Terides, M.D.; Sheehan, J.; Johnston, L.; Kayrouz, R.; Dear, R.; McEvoy, P.M.; Titov, N. Disorder-specific versus transdiagnostic and clinician-guided versus self-guided internet-delivered treatment for panic disorder and comorbid disorders: A randomized controlled trial. *J. Anxiety Disord.* **2016**, *39*, 88–102. [CrossRef]
42. Staples, L.G.; Fogliati, V.J.; Dear, B.F.; Nielssen, O.; Titov, N. Internet-delivered treatment for older adults with anxiety and depression: Implementation of the Wellbeing Plus Course in routine clinical care and comparison with research trial outcomes. *Brit. J. Psychiat. Open* **2016**, *2*, 307–313. [CrossRef]
43. Dear, B.; Staples, L.; Terides, M.; Fogliati, V.; Sheehan, J.; Johnston, L.; Kayrouz, R.; Dear, R.; McEvoy, P.; Titov, N. Transdiagnostic versus disorder-specific and clinician-guided versus self-guided internet-delivered treatment for social anxiety disorder and comorbid disorders: A randomized controlled trial. *J. Anxiety Disord.* **2016**, *42*, 30–44. [CrossRef]
44. Titov, N.; Dear, B.F.; Staples, L.G.; Terides, M.D.; Karin, E.; Sheehan, J.; Johnston, L.; Gandy, M.; Fogliati, V.J.; Wootton, B.M.; et al. Disorder-specific versus transdiagnostic and clinician-guided versus self-guided treatment for major depressive disorder and comorbid anxiety disorders: A randomized controlled trial. *J. Anxiety Disord.* **2015**, *35*, 88–102. [CrossRef]
45. Titov, N.; Fogliati, V.J.; Staples, L.G.; Gandy, M.; Johnston, L.; Wootton, B.; Nielssen, O.; Dear, B.F. Treating anxiety and depression in older adults: randomised controlled trial comparing guided v. self-guided internet-delivered cognitive–behavioural therapy. *Brit. J. Psychiat. Open* **2016**, *2*, 50–58. [CrossRef]
46. Titov, N.; Dear, B.F.; Johnston, L.; McEvoy, P.M.; Wootton, B.; Terides, M.D.; Gandy, M.; Fogliati, V.; Kayrouz, R.; Rapee, R.M. Improving adherence and clinical outcomes in self-guided internet treatment for anxiety and depression: A 12-month follow-up of a randomised controlled trial. *PLoS ONE* **2014**, *9*, e89591. [CrossRef]

47. Titov, N.; Dear, B.F.; Johnston, L.; Lorian, C.; Zou, J.; Wootton, B.; Spence, J.; McEvoy, P.M.; Rapee, R.M. Improving adherence and clinical outcomes in self-guided internet treatment for anxiety and depression: Randomised controlled trial. *PloS One* **2013**, *8*, e62873. [CrossRef]
48. Wootton, B.M.; Dear, B.F.; Johnston, L.; Terides, M.D.; Titov, N. Self-guided internet-delivered cognitive behavior therapy (iCBT) for obsessive–compulsive disorder: 12 month follow-up. *Internet Interv.* **2015**, *2*, 243–247. [CrossRef]
49. Wootton, B.M.; Dear, B.F.; Johnston, L.; Terides, M.D.; Titov, N. Remote treatment of obsessive-compulsive disorder: A randomized controlled trial. *J. Obs. Compuls. Relat. Disord.* **2013**, *2*, 375–384. [CrossRef]
50. Spence, J.; Titov, N.; Johnston, L.; Jones, M.P.; Dear, B.F.; Solley, K. Internet-based trauma-focused cognitive behavioural therapy for PTSD with and without exposure components: A randomised controlled trial. *J. Affect. Disord.* **2014**, *162*, 73–80. [CrossRef]
51. Dear, B.F.; Titov, N.; Perry, K.N.; Johnston, L.; Wootton, B.M.; Terides, M.D.; Rapee, R.M.; Hudson, J.L. The Pain Course: A randomised controlled trial of a clinician-guided Internet-delivered cognitive behaviour therapy program for managing chronic pain and emotional well-being. *Pain* **2013**, *154*, 942–950. [CrossRef]
52. Dear, B.; Staples, L.; Terides, M.; Karin, E.; Zou, J.; Johnston, L.; Gandy, M.; Fogliati, V.; Wootton, B.; McEvoy, P. Transdiagnostic versus disorder-specific and clinician-guided versus self-guided internet-delivered treatment for generalized anxiety disorder and comorbid disorders: A randomized controlled trial. *J. Anxiety Disord.* **2015**, *36*, 63–77. [CrossRef]
53. Hadjistavropoulos, H.D. *Online Therapy Unit Outcome Report 2013-2017*; University of Regina: Regina, SK, Canada, 2018.
54. Hadjistavropoulos, H.D.; Faller, Y.N.; Klatt, A.; Nugent, M.N.; Dear, B.F.; Titov, N. Patient Perspectives on Strengths and Challenges of Therapist-Assisted Internet-Delivered Cognitive Behaviour Therapy: Using the Patient Voice to Improve Care. *Community Ment. Health J.* **2018**, *54*, 944–950. [CrossRef]
55. Hadjistavropoulos, H.D.; Schneider, L.H.; Mehta, S.; Karin, E.; Dear, B.F.; Titov, N. Preference trial of internet-delivered cognitive behaviour therapy comparing standard weekly versus optional weekly therapist support. *J. Anxiety Disord.* **2019**, *63*, 51–60. [CrossRef]
56. Titov, N.; Schofield, C.; Staples, L.; Dear, B.F.; Nielssen, O. A comparison of Indigenous and non-Indigenous users of MindSpot: An Australian digital mental health service. *Australas. Psychiatry* **2018**, *27*, 352–357. [CrossRef]
57. Hadjistavropoulos, H.D.; Thompson, M.J.; Klein, B.; Austin, D.W. Dissemination of Therapist-Assisted Internet Cognitive Behaviour Therapy: Development and Open Pilot Study of a Workshop. *Cog. Behav. Ther.* **2012**, *41*, 230–240. [CrossRef]
58. Hadjistavropoulos, H.D.; Gullickson, K.M.; Schneider, L.H.; Dear, B.F.; Titov, N. Development of the Internet-Delivered Cognitive Behaviour Therapy Undesirable Therapist Behaviours Scale (ICBT-UTBS). *Internet Interv.* **2019**. [CrossRef]
59. Andersson, G.; Cuijpers, P.; Carlbring, P.; Riper, H.; Hedman, E. Guided Internet-based vs. face-to-face cognitive behavior therapy for psychiatric and somatic disorders: A systematic review and meta-analysis. *World Psychiatry* **2014**, *13*, 288–295 [CrossRef]
60. Hadjistavropoulos, H.D.; Pugh, N.E.; Hesser, H.; Andersson, G. Therapeutic Alliance in Internet-Delivered Cognitive Behaviour Therapy for Depression or Generalized Anxiety. *Clin. Psychol. Psychother.* **2016**, *24*, 451–461. [CrossRef]
61. Hadjistavropoulos, H.D.; Schneider, L.H.; Klassen, K.; Dear, B.F.; Titov, N. Development and evaluation of a scale assessing therapist fidelity to guidelines for delivering therapist-assisted Internet-delivered cognitive behaviour therapy. *Cogn. Behav. Ther.* **2018**, *47*, 447–461. [CrossRef]
62. Hatfield, D.R.; Ogles, B.M. The Use of Outcome Measures by Psychologists in Clinical Practice. *Prof. Psychol. Res. Pract.* **2004**, *35*, 485–491. [CrossRef]
63. Boswell, J.F.; Kraus, D.R.; Miller, S.D.; Lambert, M.J. Implementing routine outcome monitoring in clinical practice: Benefits, challenges, and solutions. *Psychother. Res.* **2015**, *25*, 6–19. [CrossRef]
64. Jensen-Doss, A.; Haimes, E.M.B.; Smith, A.M.; Lyon, A.R.; Lewis, C.C.; Stanick, C.F.; Hawley, K.M. Monitoring Treatment Progress and Providing Feedback is Viewed Favorably but Rarely Used in Practice. *Adm. Policy Ment. Health Ment. Health Serv. Res.* **2018**, *45*, 48–61. [CrossRef]
65. Australian Government. *National Standards for Mental Health Services*; Department of Health, Ed.; Australian Government: Canberra, Australian, 2010.

66. Commonwealth of Australia. *Quality Framework for Telephone Counselling and Internet-based Support Services*; Department of Health and Ageing, Australian Government: Canberra, Australian, 2009.
67. Hadjistavropoulos, H.D.; Pugh, N.E.; Hesser, H.; Andersson, G. Predicting Response to Therapist-Assisted Internet-Delivered Cognitive Behavior Therapy for Depression or Anxiety Within an Open Dissemination Trial. *Behav. Ther.* **2016**, *47*, 155–165. [CrossRef]
68. Mental Health Commission of Canada. *E-Mental Health in Canada: Transforming the Mental Health System Using Technology*; Mental Health Commission of Canada: Ottawa, ON, Canada, 2014.
69. National Mental Health Service Planning Framework. Available online: https://nmhspf.org.au/ (accessed on 27 June 2019).
70. Urech, A.; Krieger, T.; Möseneder, L.; Biaggi, A.; Vincent, A.; Poppe, C.; Meyer, B.; Riper, H.; Berger, T. A patient post hoc perspective on advantages and disadvantages of blended cognitive behaviour therapy for depression: A qualitative content analysis. *Psychother. Res.* **2018**, *31*, 1–13. [CrossRef]
71. Mol, M.; Dozeman, E.; Provoost, S.; van Schaik, A.; Riper, H.; Smit, J.H. Behind the Scenes of Online Therapeutic Feedback in Blended Therapy for Depression: Mixed-Methods Observational Study. *J. Med Internet Res.* **2018**, *20*, e174. [CrossRef]
72. Erbe, D.; Eichert, H.C.; Riper, H.; Ebert, D.D. Blending face-to-face and internet-based interventions for the treatment of mental disorders in adults: Systematic review. *J. Med Internet Res.* **2017**, *19*, e306. [CrossRef]
73. Mathiasen, K.; Andersen, T.E.; Riper, H.; Kleiboer, A.A.M.; Roessler, K.K. Blended CBT versus face-to-face CBT: A randomised non-inferiority trial. *BMC Psychiatry* **2016**, *16*, 432. [CrossRef]
74. Kleiboer, A.; Smit, J.; Bosmans, J.; Ruwaard, J.; Andersson, G.; Topooco, N.; Berger, T.; Krieger, T.; Botella, C.; Baños, R.; et al. European COMPARative Effectiveness research on blended Depression treatment versus treatment-as-usual (E-COMPARED): Study protocol for a randomized controlled, non-inferiority trial in eight European countries. *Trials* **2016**, *17*, 387. [CrossRef]
75. Soucy, J.N.; Owens, V.A.M.; Hadjistavropoulos, H.D.; Dirkse, D.A.; Dear, B.F. Educating patients about Internet-delivered cognitive behaviour therapy: Perceptions among treatment seekers and non-treatment seekers before and after viewing an educational video. *Internet Interv.* **2016**, *6*, 57–63. [CrossRef]
76. Choi, I.; Zou, J.; Titov, N.; Dear, B.F.; Li, S.; Johnston, L.; Andrews, G.; Hunt, C. Culturally attuned Internet treatment for depression amongst Chinese Australians: A randomised controlled trial. *J. Affect. Disord.* **2012**, *136*, 459–68. [CrossRef]
77. Kayrouz, R.; Dear, B.F.; Kayrouz, B.; Karin, E.; Gandy, M.; Titov, N. Meta-analysis of the efficacy and acceptability of cognitive-behavioural therapy for Arab adult populations experiencing anxiety, depression or post-traumatic stress disorder. *Cogn. Behav. Ther.* **2018**, *47*, 412–430. [CrossRef]
78. Kayrouz, R.; Dear, B.F.; Karin, E.; Fogliati, V.J.; Titov, N. A pilot study of a clinician-guided internet-delivered cognitive behavioural therapy for anxiety and depression among Arabs in Australia, presented in both English and Arabic languages. *Internet Interv.* **2016**, *5*, 5–11. [CrossRef]
79. American Psychological Association, Guidelines for the Practice of Telepsychology. *Am. Psychol.* **2013**, *68*, 791–800. [CrossRef]
80. Association of Canadian Psychology Regulatory Organizations. *Model Standards for Telepsychology Service Delivery*; ACPRO: Saskatchewan, Canadian, 2011; pp. 1–3.
81. Royal Australian and New Zealand College of Psychiatrists. *Benefits of E-Mental Health Treatments and Interventions*; RANZCP: Melbourne, Australian, 2019.
82. Available online: http://www.emhprac.org.au/e-MentalHealthinPractice (accessed on 26 June 2019).
83. Ruwaard, J.; Kok, R. Wild West eHealth: Time to hold our horses? *Eur. Health Psychol.* **2015**, *17*, 45–49.
84. Rozental, A.; Andersson, G.; Boettcher, J.; Ebert, D.D.; Cuijpers, P.; Knaevelsrud, C.; Ljótsson, B.; Kaldo, V.; Titov, N.; Carlbring, P. Consensus statement on defining and measuring negative effects of Internet interventions. *Internet Interv.* **2014**, *1*, 12–19. [CrossRef]

Journal of
Clinical Medicine

MDPI

Article

Why Uptake of Blended Internet-Based Interventions for Depression Is Challenging: A Qualitative Study on Therapists' Perspectives

Mayke Mol [1,2,*], Claire van Genugten [1,2], Els Dozeman [1,2], Digna J. F. van Schaik [1,2], Stasja Draisma [1,2], Heleen Riper [1,2,3,4] and Jan H. Smit [1,2]

1 Department of Research and Innovation, GGZ inGeest, Specialized Mental Health Care, 1081 Amsterdam, The Netherlands; c.genugten@ggzingeest.nl (C.v.G.); e.dozeman@ggzingeest.nl (E.D.); a.schaik@ggzingeest.nl (D.J.F.v.S.); s.draisma@ggzingeest.nl (S.D.); h.riper@vu.nl (H.R.); jh.smit@ggzingeest.nl (J.H.S.)

2 Department of Psychiatry, Amsterdam Public Health Research Institute, VU University Medical Center, 1081 Amsterdam, The Netherlands

3 Department of Clinical, Neuro and Developmental Psychology, Clinical Psychology Section, Vrije Universiteit Amsterdam and the Amsterdam Public Health Research Institute, 1081 Amsterdam, The Netherlands

4 Telepsychiatry and E-Mental Health, Department of Clinical Research, University of Southern Denmark, 5000 Odense, Denmark

* Correspondence: m.mol@ggzingeest.nl; Tel.: +31-(0)20-788-4624

Received: 23 November 2019; Accepted: 20 December 2019; Published: 30 December 2019

Abstract: (1) Background: Blended cognitive behavioral therapy (bCBT; online and face-to-face sessions) seems a promising alternative alongside regular face-to-face CBT depression treatment in specialized mental health care organizations. Therapists are key in the uptake of bCBT. This study focuses on therapists' perspectives on usability, satisfaction, and factors that promote or hinder the use of bCBT in routine practice; (2) Methods: Three focus groups ($n = 8$, $n = 7$, $n = 6$) and semi-structured in-depth interviews ($n = 15$) were held throughout the Netherlands. Beforehand, the participating therapists ($n = 36$) completed online questionnaires on usability and satisfaction. Interviews were analyzed by thematic analysis; (3) Results: Therapists found the usability sufficient and were generally satisfied with providing bCBT. The thematic analysis showed three main themes on promoting and hindering factors: (1) therapists' needs regarding bCBT uptake, (2) therapists' role in motivating patients for bCBT, and (3) therapists' experiences with bCBT; (4) Conclusions: Overall, therapists were positive; bCBT can be offered by all CBT-trained therapists and future higher uptake is expected. Especially the pre-set structure of bCBT was found beneficial for both therapists and patients. Nevertheless, therapists did not experience promised time-savings—rather, the opposite. Besides, there are still teething problems and therapeutic shortcomings that need improvement in order to motivate therapists to use bCBT.

Keywords: cognitive behavioral therapy; blended treatment; depressive disorder; implementation; therapists' perspective; routine care

1. Background

Face-to-face (FtF) cognitive behavioral therapy (CBT) is an evidence-based treatment for depression [1]. According to international guidelines, CBT is a standard option for treating patients with depression in specialized mental health care [2]. Unfortunately, patient access to CBT is hindered by several barriers such as perceived personal stigma, costs, long waiting lists, and limited availability of licensed therapists [3,4]. It seems therefore promising to offer CBT with the support of technology and without the FtF sessions, thereby potentially reducing therapists' time and costs due to increased involvement of patients themselves. In Internet-based cognitive behavioral therapy (iCBT), treatment access can be improved to offer CBT on an online platform. This would help reduce stigma, waiting lists, and costs, since patients can work through sessions at their own pace, in their own time, and therapist time is lessened. It has been shown that iCBT, especially with online therapist guidance, has good clinical effects for patients with depression [5,6].

In geographically dispersed countries like Canada and Australia, online clinics have successfully reached many patients through iCBT (e.g., Mindspot Clinic, Online Therapy Unit) [7]. In the Netherlands, iCBT, with guidance at a distance, has been offered by Interapy for more than two decades (www.interapy.nl). This mental health care organization (MHO) was founded as an online therapy center and provides specialized online evidenced-based care for among other thing depression, trauma and panic disorder. Other MHO's, where face-to-face treatments are the standard, also are implementing iCBT to improve patient access and make treatments more cost-efficient. However, iCBT uptake in MHOs is limited. This might be partly because therapists perceive iCBT to be limited in crisis situations, ineligible for severe depressive symptoms, and having a one-size fits all approach [8,9]. In addition, given the relatively high density of mental health services, the need for iCBT in the Netherlands may differ from elsewhere.

Blended CBT, a new format of iCBT, which has been recently adopted by MHOs in routine care systems in the Netherlands, could address the limitations since online sessions are combined with FtF sessions in a single, integrated, standardized CBT treatment protocol [10]. bCBT aims to improve both quality of care and cost-efficacy by replacing a portion of the FtF sessions with online sessions [11,12]. Through reducing the number of FtF sessions, therapists' time is saved, they can potentially treat more patients, and waiting lists can be shortened. In addition, within the online platform, therapist contact is extended beyond the FtF sessions by online communication. A number of studies have shown that bCBT can be effective in treating patients with depression [13–15]. However, similarly to iCBT in MHOs, the uptake of bCBT by therapists and patients is limited as it has not yet been implemented across the board in MHOs in the Netherlands and elsewhere [16].

The gap between promising research findings and the limited iCBT and bCBT uptake in routine practice was one of the reasons behind the European MasterMind project, designed to increase and evaluate uptake and implementation of Internet-based interventions in ten European countries (www.mastermind-project.eu) [17]. In MasterMind there was a specific focus on therapists' perspectives, as they play a substantial role in the uptake of iCBT and bCBT. And besides, studies concerning therapists' perspectives in routine practice are scarce [18].

In a qualitative study in Germany, several barriers and facilitators were identified based on the perspectives of therapists (n = 5) providing bCBT alongside a randomized controlled study [19]. Key issues varied from problematic platform technology to an unclear concept of embedding bCBT in the mental health care system. Despite the barriers, therapists viewed bCBT as an adequate treatment option for patients with depression. To build on this, more in-depth knowledge on therapists' perspectives in specialized routine care could contribute to optimizing uptake of bCBT, as the therapists' workflow and patient-related factors are more complex in daily practice than in research settings.

The objective of this qualitative study was to investigate therapists' perspectives in routine care when transitioning to using bCBT as an alternative alongside CBT for patients with depression within outpatient specialized mental health care settings in the Netherlands. To increase insight into the factors that influence uptake of bCBT in routine care, the following questions were answered using data triangulation [20] in the context of questionnaires, focus groups, and semi-structured interviews with therapists:

- What are the therapist perspectives on bCBT usability (e.g., perceived ease of use of the platform)?
- How satisfied are therapists with offering bCBT (e.g., overall satisfaction with bCBT)?
- What are the therapist perspectives on factors that promote or hinder the use of bCBT in daily practice (e.g., training, patient eligibility, safety)?

2. Methods

2.1. Therapists

Therapists were (CBT trained) psychologists, mental health nurses, or psychiatrists working at seven MHOs where bCBT had been implemented. To be included in the study, therapists had to be trained in the use of the online platform prior to or during the study period.

The therapists were employed at small (200 registrations for depression per year) to large private-non-profit MHOs (5000 depression registrations per year) spread across the Netherlands. All organizations had bCBT available on a platform from the same large commercial provider (Minddistrict; www.minddistrict.com)—most since 2014. MHOs provided bCBT training to (all or a part of) their therapists either 'in-house' or externally by the provider, or via online training. The estimated duration of the training varied from four hours to two days. MHO's stimulated therapists in different ways for bCBT (e.g., by setting bCBT targets or by special blended consultation hours), however therapists could make their own decision about the treatment of choice.

2.2. Recruitment

Through other users of the Minddistrict platform and personal contacts of the authors, 10 MHOs were invited to be part of the study because they implemented an online platform into routine care. One MHO withdrew because it ceased to exist, another MHO was too busy with ongoing other projects and trials, and one MHO switched to a different platform provider and needed time to explore other providers. In total, seven MHOs participated.

Therapists were identified through team managers, and other specially members of different teams, appointed by the manager of the MHOs. Therapists for focus groups or in-depth interviews were purposively sampled to cover diversity of use and experience with bCBT, age, professional background, and geographic region. First, therapists from two MHOs were invited to participate in a focus group. The focus groups were held within the context of the European implementation project MasterMind. The MasterMind project ran from March 2014 to February 2017. For a more detailed description, see the study protocol of the MasterMind study in the Netherlands [18]. In total, 3 focus groups were held with 21 participants.

Second, to add more depth to the topics discussed in the focus groups, complementary semi-structured individual interviews were held with therapists (who had not participated in the focus groups) from seven MHOs. After 15 interviews, no new information or themes were brought up and data saturation was reached. Two weeks prior to the focus group and interviews, all participating therapists received an informed consent form and questionnaires were used to gather information on therapist demographics, satisfaction, and usability of bCBT via a secure online survey tool (Survalyzer; www.survalyzer.com). Figure 1 provides an outline of the study.

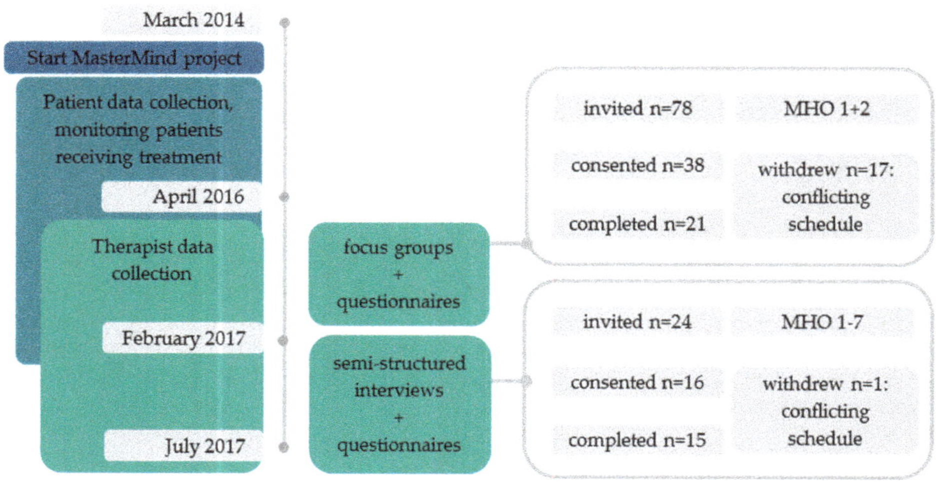

Figure 1. Study outline.

2.3. Intervention

Therapists worked with an integrated bCBT protocol in which FtF and online sessions were alternated. The blended protocol for depression mostly consisted of 10 online sessions. These were supported by FtF sessions (for mild or moderate depression 5 FtF sessions every two weeks; and for (very) severe depression 10 to 11 weekly FtF-sessions). bCBT started and ended with a FtF session. Therapists could individualize the protocol to the patient's needs by repeating and/or skipping online sessions. More detailed information about the protocol can be found elsewhere [21].

Patients could be offered bCBT if (1) they were aged 18 years or older; (2) had a mild, moderate, or severe depression as a primary diagnosis according to the therapist; and (3) were indicated for cognitive behavioral treatment for depression following routine secondary mental health care procedures. Exclusion criteria were (1) not having a valid email address and a computer with Internet access and (2) not having adequate Dutch language skills (both verbal and written).

Therapists had access to the (Minddistrict) platform through a dashboard, which showed treatment sessions, including homework assignments, and had optional functions for a patient diary and depressive symptom questionnaires. The role of the therapists was to monitor the patients' online progress and to provide patients with personalized written feedback to homework assignments after each completed online session. Therapists could additionally communicate through a message function on the platform about practical issues (e.g., upcoming appointments, reminders, or questions about assignments). The safety of the platform was guaranteed by meeting the European requirements for certified data security [22].

2.4. Data Collection

2.4.1. Questionnaires

The 10 items of the System Usability Scale measured perceived usability (SUS) [23]. The SUS is a validated questionnaire for evaluating usability of Internet-based interventions as perceived by therapists and showed a good reliability (omega coefficient = 0.91) [24]. It is unofficially translated in Dutch [25]. The score for the total score range from 0 to 100. A score above the cut-off of 68 is considered to be above average [26]. The Client Satisfaction Questionnaire-3 measured satisfaction with bCBT (CSQ-3), is officially translated to Dutch [27] and was adapted to therapists (e.g., CSQ1 = To what extent has the bCBT intervention met your needs in treating depressed patients?). The CSQ showed good reliability (McDonald omega = 0.95) and validity in a sample of Internet-based depression intervention users [28].

2.4.2. Focus Group Interviews

To identify relevant therapist factors in bCBT uptake, dimensions of the RE-AIM framework (Reach, Effectiveness, Adoption, Implementation, Maintenance) [29], the MAST framework (Model for assessment of telemedicine) [30], and the normalization process theory [31] were used to build and structure the focus group topic list (see File S1 in Supplementary Materials). The main predetermined themes were: patient and therapist factors, barriers and facilitators, satisfaction and usability. The focus group was pilot tested with a moderator and three participants who acted as therapists to refine the topic list and time management. Key questions were presented on a PowerPoint presentation during the therapist focus groups. Via a mobile voting system (Sendsteps; www.sendsteps.com), participants could give their opinion on certain questions and statements in order to stimulate discussion. Discussions were moderated by senior researcher and co-author S.D. with experience in conducting focus groups. They were assisted by researcher and first-author M.M. The focus groups were audio-recorded. The duration of the focus groups was 100–115 min and they took place at the participating MHOs. To increase validity, a transcript of each focus group was sent to each participant for feedback.

2.4.3. Semi-Structured In-Depth Interviews

In semi-structured interviews, therapists were asked individually to reflect on the same topics as in the focus groups to further explore personal experiences. In addition, questions were added based on interview guides from previous research [19,32,33] as well as outcomes of the focus groups; there were slightly different questions for therapists with and without experience in providing bCBT for depression (see File S2 and S3 for the topic lists in Supplementary Materials). After 10 interviews, 3 additional topics were added since these seemed relevant to therapists (e.g., experience with writing online feedback, preferred ratio of online versus FtF sessions and preferred starting point for introduction of online platform). Interviews were conducted by two researchers (M.M. and C.v.G.). The interviews lasted 35–90 min. Most interviews were held at the MHOs (n = 10); five were conducted by telephone for practical reasons. The interviews were audio-recorded. An interview transcript was sent to each participant for respondent validation.

2.5. Data Analyses

Descriptive analyses (frequencies, means, and percentages) of the quantitative data (demographics of therapists, perceived satisfaction, and usability) were performed with SPSS, version 22.0 (IBM Corp. Armonk, NY, USA). Atlas-ti.7 software was used for qualitative analysis (version 7 and 8, Scientific Software Development GmbH. Berlin, Germany).

Focus groups and semi-structured in-depth interview transcripts were concurrently analyzed with thematic analysis techniques guided by the following steps [34]: (1) familiarization with the data; (re-)reading of the transcripts and field notes; (2) generating initial codes; developing a codebook; (3) searching for (sub)themes; identifying broad topics; refining codebook; (4) reviewing the (sub)themes; (5) defining and naming (sub)themes; and (6) reporting. Anonymity was assured by using code numbers instead of names. Each sentence in the transcripts could contain multiple codes, and concurrent sentences of the same thematic code could be conjoined into one unit.

In the results section, therapist' quotes were selected to illustrate the essence of a (sub)theme. The statements reflected perspectives from both focus groups and interviews. We chose to pool these sources as similar topics were discussed and no overlap existed between the therapists who participated in the focus groups and interviews. Both contributed to a more comprehensive understanding of therapists' perspectives. When a perspective concerned a minority of therapists, patients, or other therapists within the participating organizations, this is explicitly mentioned.

To ensure reliability, agreement on codes and concepts between members of the research team was sought. Researchers M.M., C.v.G., and S.D. coded 4 interviews together until acceptable agreement (Fleiss kappa >0.50) was reached [35]. The remaining interviews were divided equally between researchers M.M. and C.v.G. Data collection process, data analysis, and any interim findings, as well as quality and methodological aspects, were discussed in the research group continuously.

2.6. Ethical Issues

The study was approved by the Medical Ethics Committee of the VU medical center, Amsterdam. They confirmed that the Medical Research Involving Human Subjects Act does not apply (registration number 2014.580) because therapists in this study were not required to follow certain procedures on behalf of the research (no randomization), and routine practice was followed. An internal scientific research committee approved the research proposal.

3. Results

Table 1 presents therapist demographics and experience. With respect to distribution of experience with bCBT for depression, 42% of the therapists had considerable bCBT experience (providing bCBT 5 to 20 times or more), 42% had little experience (providing bCBT 1 to 4 times), and 17% had no experience.

Table 1. Therapist demographics and experience.

Therapist Demographics	$n = 36$
Gender, female, n (%)	29 (81)
Age in years, mean (SD; range)	38 (9.5; 24–60)
Professional background, n (%)	
Licensed psychologists	20 (56)
Psychologists in training under supervision for health care psychologists	5 (14)
Mental health nurses	5 (14)
Other (e.g., psychiatrists, prevention workers)	6 (16)
Professional experience, n (%)	
0–2 years	3 (8)
3–4 years	8 (22)
5–9 years	10 (27)
10 years or more	15 (42)
bCBT depression treatment experience, n (%)	
0 times	6 (17)
1–4 times	15 (42)
5–9 times	8 (22)
10–19 times	2 (6)
20 or more times	5 (14)

3.1. bCBT Usability

The mean SUS total score was 69.5 (SD 11.1; range 42.5–90.0). This score indicates sufficient usability of the bCBT platform. In the focus groups and interviews, therapists indicated that the usability had evolved over time. However, the current technical status still needs further improvement. For some, platform usability was a barrier to providing bCBT because many extra actions were required (e.g., logging in, finding the module, setting up the sessions). In addition, there was no integration with other (administrative) computer systems that therapists frequently use (e.g., electronic medical records). Moreover, therapists felt hampered by the lack of knowhow and of a clear overview of all the functions and were unsure how to adapt the protocol. For example, it was unclear to them how to add sessions focused on panic attacks. Some therapists felt the platform usability was complicated and not intuitive. Unexpected updates by the provider did not improve this. For therapists with little bCBT experience, the concern that they would be unable to assist patients with technical problems was also a major barrier. In addition, therapists had negative experiences with contacting the helpdesk (e.g., lack of expertise): "I trained myself to not contact the helpdesk anymore" (T23, experienced).

3.2. bCBT Satisfaction

On the CSQ-3, 77% of therapists stated that bCBT met all or almost all their needs; 94% were overall very or mostly satisfied with bCBT; and 97% would recommend bCBT in the future to their patients. Interestingly, in the focus groups and interviews, the opinions of other therapists about satisfaction were divided: some thought that most therapists were generally satisfied, others said: "I also think that therapists are rather dissatisfied. bCBT isn't used on a large scale. This means they must be dissatisfied, otherwise they would use it" (T28, no/little experience).

Most of the therapists indicated that they would like to use bCBT in the future, but this depended on several preconditions that needed to be addressed: platform usability, their current work routine, and more guidelines on how to use bCBT.

3.3. Factors That Promote or Hinder Uptake of bCBT

Regardless of the amount of bCBT experience, therapists were in favor of bCBT. Their views on the factors that promoted or hindered the use of bCBT in daily practice were structured along main themes identified in thematic analysis: (1) therapists' needs regarding bCBT uptake, (2) therapists' role in motivating patients for bCBT, and (3) therapists' experiences with bCBT (See Table 2 for main and subthemes).

Table 2. Therapists' blended cognitive behavioral therapy (bCBT) uptake in routine practice, main themes, and subthemes.

Theme (1) Therapists' Needs Regarding bCBT Uptake	Theme (2) Therapists' Role in Motivating Patients for bCBT	Theme (3) Therapists' Experiences with bCBT
Therapist training Therapist motivation Therapist readiness for uptake	Informing patients Patient eligibility Patient resistance	Effectiveness for depression Positive effects Negative effects Treatment protocol Therapeutic relationship Online feedback skills Drop-out and safety

3.3.1. Theme (1) Therapists' Needs Regarding bCBT Uptake

This theme addresses factors related to therapists' needs in providing bCBT to patients with depression. The identified subthemes were: therapist training, therapist motivation, and therapist readiness for uptake (Table 3).

Table 3. Theme (1) Therapists' needs regarding bCBT uptake, subthemes, influencing factors, and illustrative quotes.

Subtheme	Influencing Factors	Illustrative Quotes
Therapist training	(+) sufficient to learn the technical aspects	*"It is nice to have learned beforehand where all the buttons are and what the possibilities are."* (T11, no/little experience)
	(−) lack of therapeutic content and guidelines in the training	*"I miss therapeutic content in the training and the qualifications for the therapists to work with it."* (T25, experience)
	(−) training alone is not enough for uptake in daily practice	*"There is one training and then you're released with the notion: 'now you can manage everything'."* (T7, experience)

Table 3. *Cont.*

Subtheme	Influencing Factors	Illustrative Quotes
	(−) lack of ongoing support	*"There is a lack of time to delve into it, it should be facilitated better and not end with a single training."* (T14, no/little experience)
Therapist motivation	(−) demotivated therapists	*"What bothers me most when it comes to blended is that it has been made mandatory, mainly because we've to meet a certain percentage of blended treatments."* (T34, experience)
	(+) motivated therapists	*"If you are a psychologist, and you are interested in your profession, you should just use it."* (T9, experience)
	(−/+) undecided therapists	*"You have to get out of your comfort zone to discover what the added value of blended is."* (T31, no/little experience)
Therapist readiness for uptake	(−) small select group uses bCBT on a regular basis	*"When I look at my team, it seems only one person is trained, I don't really hear others talk about it."* (T36, experience)
	(+) expected to grow in future	*"I'd like to use blended in the future, but first I'd like more ideas on how to use it* (T6, no/little experience)
	(−/+) making bCBT mandatory	*"I once heard that you need a certain percentage of online contacts—that would work for me."* (T2, experience)

Note. (−) factor that influenced the bCBT uptake negatively, (+) factor that influenced the bCBT uptake positively, (−/+) factor that influenced the bCBT uptake positively and negatively.

Therapist Training

Most therapists found the training formats sufficient for providing bCBT. The focus in the training formats was primarily targeted at technical aspects and less at therapeutic content. The therapists reported that they needed more guidelines and tools for providing online feedback, to keep patients engaged and to prevent them from deviating from the protocol. The training formats in their current form were probably sufficient for the 'early adopters' but less suited for therapists with limited computer skills, the older generation, or new graduates.

Moreover, undergoing training alone was not enough. Therapists found it difficult to familiarize themselves with the platform, and integrate bCBT into existing systems and into their daily workflow. Time constraints were the most frequently cited barrier for uptake of bCBT. This was mainly due to a high caseload. Plus, therapists felt that the implementation ceased after the training was provided, and that the training was fragmented and was introduced too suddenly. Consequently, some organizations offered therapists a special consultation hour or extra training day. Yet, only a select group of motivated therapists turned up at these events. In order to integrate bCBT into their work routine, therapists needed more ongoing technical and content support in the form of supervision or peer review.

Above all, every qualified therapist was considered able to provide blended treatment, mostly because bCBT was perceived as being very similar to regular CBT. However, they also believed that therapist qualifications and professional background have so far been overlooked. They felt sufficient knowledge and professional experience of CBT should be a criterion for being trained in bCBT.

Therapist Motivation

Therapists in this study were motivated for bCBT. Their colleagues could roughly be divided into three groups based on their motivation: demotivated therapists, motivated therapists, and an inexperienced group that needed more motivation.

Therapists estimated that about half of their therapist colleagues were not motivated for bCBT. They thought that perceived pressure from the MHOs and health care insurance companies worked counterproductively. Other reasons were varied. Some thought that a number of colleagues tended to resist every innovation implemented by the organization. For others, the reasons were fear-based:

(1) fear that technology will eventually take over, (2) fear of losing contact when a patient is inactive on the platform, (3) fear of not offering patients the amount of help they need, and/or (4) fear that they would do something wrong or would come across as unprofessional towards patients. A specific group of therapists, who were enthusiastic at the start but due to negative experiences with (other/outdated/unguided) Internet-based interventions, lost interest or became sceptical about the clinical effects of bCBT. This was mainly due to technical issues and higher patient drop-out rates.

Motivated therapists were described as being younger, having affinity with technology, and being interested in innovations in their field. Not every therapist was open to the idea of bCBT in the beginning, but some adjusted their view based on (positive) experiences.

Non-experienced therapists were mainly profiled as lacking computer skills, having technical skills insecurities, and belonging to an older generation with a traditional view on therapy. Interestingly, it was stated multiple times that many therapists were open to bCBT and also were capable of delivering it, but had reservations that first needed to be addressed. On top of a strong preference for FtF treatment over bCBT, there are thought to be many therapists to whom the possibilities of bCBT were unknown or remained unclear. They were often unaware of its added value or of research findings. For them, the need for blended did not come from within. However, even though there might be many reasons not to provide bCBT, therapists believed that only a small proportion are truly resistant to it.

Therapist Readiness for Uptake

Though most therapists received training on the back of an organization-wide roll-out, a number observed that only a select group used bCBT on a daily base. To some, this was related to readiness for uptake: the implementation of bCBT in routine care is considered to be at an early, transitional stage. Although it might be too innovative for therapists and patients, they believed that a change in perception toward bCBT will take place, and that readiness would increase as more patients start asking for bCBT.

There was disagreement with respect to making bCBT obligatory or not. For some, it would feed resistance toward bCBT and fuel the suspicion that bCBT was solely implemented for financial reasons. Others believed that every therapist should 'just use it' or at least try it. It was also felt that treatment should be 'blended, unless a therapist has limited computer skills, or a different therapeutic background or interest'. Most therapists stressed that for them, the precondition that blended stays blended is of great importance, because of the fear that MHOs in the future might gradually transition to online CBT.

3.3.2. Theme (2) Therapists' Role in Motivating Patients for bCBT

The second theme concerns the role of therapists in motivating patients with depression to use bCBT. The identified subthemes were: informing patients, patient eligibility, and patient resistance (Table 4).

Table 4. Theme (2) Therapists' role in motivating patients for bCBT, subthemes, influencing factors, and illustrative quotes.

Subtheme	Influencing Factors	Illustrative Quotes
Informing patients	(−) difficult to motivate some patients	*"Sometimes there is so much going on, which leads me to inform patients in an insecure or doubtful way, that makes them say 'no, I don't want that'."* (T35, no/little experience)
	(−) room for improvement	*"I think that therapists should 'sell' or promote bCBT more with patients."* (T15, experience)

Table 4. *Cont.*

Subtheme	Influencing Factors	Illustrative Quotes
Patient eligibility	(−) eligible patient unknown	*"It is difficult to assess for whom it is eligible. Sometimes someone who grew up with computers says, 'oh no, not for me', and then a 65-year old says 'nice, let's do it'."* (T10, experience)
	(−/+) discussion on comorbidity/complexity/ depression severity	*"I imagine that blended is less suitable for more complex cases. But if I consider what I have in my caseload now, I think it should be doable."* (T5, no/little experience)
	(+) eligibility bCBT = eligibility CBT	*"In principle everyone is eligible for bCBT. I rarely think that it's not an option."* (T7, experience)
Patient resistance	(−) unclear image, too demanding, not enough, negative past experiences	*"Patients don't have a good image of bCBT. In their view it's more like an online questionnaire than a complete module, 'I've already answered those questions … '."* (T9, experience)
	(+) patient demand expected to increase in the future	*"I think it will make an essential difference if patients ask for it. That's just a matter of time'."* (T1, no/little experience)

Note. (−) factor that influenced the bCBT uptake negatively, (+) factor that influenced the bCBT uptake positively, (−/+) factor that influenced the bCBT uptake positively and negatively.

Informing Patients

Many therapists had difficulties informing patients about bCBT for various reasons. Reasons given included the following: they were convinced that patients preferred FtF contact; blended was considered too demanding for patients; or they thought that patients would not need bCBT. Therapists thought that more effort could be put into convincing patients since the manner in which bCBT is offered could influence patients' reactions.

Therapists found it a disadvantage that patients did not ask for bCBT or lacked a clear idea of what blended entails. Therefore, therapists believed it could be facilitating to offer it with enthusiasm, to explain the added value: 'patients can do more in their own time, there is more information to their disposal, and they have more opportunities to practice, all in a secure environment'. It was indicated that there is a lot of room for improvement when it comes to informing patients. It helped, for example, if patients knew that it is their own therapist who communicates with them on the platform. In addition, to increase uptake, therapists should not offer it as a treatment option, but as the standard approach to treating depression. Some therapists offered blended as something extra, whereas others showed patients the platform during intake to facilitate the switch to the platform at a later point during treatment.

Patient Eligibility

Experienced therapists mentioned that the criteria for bCBT were very similar to the criteria for CBT. No specific patient bCBT profile or type existed; eligibility was found to be person specific, not predictable and sometimes even very surprising. Therapists with little or no bCBT experience gave many different criteria for patient eligibility, which were predominantly based on perceptions.

A contributing factor to difficulties with informing patients was the unknown typology of the eligible bCBT patient. Stated criteria for perceived non-eligibility were extensive: lack of computer skills, preference for FtF treatment, fear of failure, lack of illness insight, low cognitive capacities, limited language skills, insecure home environment, psychotic symptoms, suicidal ideation, personality disorder, trauma, and complex or severe depressive symptoms. Perceived eligible patient criteria were less elaborate: young age, having children, being employed, and mild to moderate depressive symptoms.

Two interesting discussions took place about patient eligibility. Therapists disagreed about patients who, besides depression, had autism, avoidance issues, limited social contacts, poor concentration skills, or had undergone CBT for depression in the past. Some therapists observed that these factors prevented patients from engaging with bCBT, whereas others experienced that these factors made bCBT explicitly eligible for these patients as well. Another point of discussion was the severity of the depressive symptoms. Some therapists thought that bCBT was suitable for patients with complex, severe problems, while others did not: it would be harder to activate them than patients with less complex and more moderate symptoms. They would need more tools and explanations than bCBT can possibly offer them.

Patient Resistance

Several reasons for patient resistance toward bCBT were observed: unclear bCBT image, misfit with the traditional image of therapy among patients who had CBT in the past, fear of not receiving the right amount of help, and thinking that the online component was too demanding. Therapists' found that some patients were more difficult to motivate because they were inclined to generalize negative experiences with previous Internet-based treatments (often unguided treatments in primary care) to all other Internet-based interventions. However, most therapists, especially the experienced ones, thought the vast majority of patients were positive about bCBT when offered. Most therapists agreed that patient demand will increase in the future.

3.3.3. Theme (3) Therapists' Experiences with bCBT

Within this theme, experiences with providing bCBT in routine care are discussed. The identified subthemes were: effectiveness for depression, positive effects, negative effects, treatment format, therapeutic relationship, online feedback skills, drop-out, and safety (see Table 5).

Table 5. Theme (3) Therapists' experiences with bCBT, subthemes, influencing factors, and illustrative quotes.

Subtheme	Influencing Factors	Illustrative Quotes
Effectiveness for depression	(+) effectiveness bCBT = effectiveness of CBT	*"It is CBT in another format, it's not suddenly a different treatment."* (T29, experience)
Positive effects	(+) containing therapist drift	*"I don't skip things. With bCBT, I think that I am much more thorough than without."* (T29, experience)
	(+) making other diagnosis or problems more easily visible	*"You notice much sooner if a patient has difficulties adhering to therapy, whether or not they are doing the work. This becomes clearer faster than in a FtF session."* (T1, no/little experience)
	(+) helps to remember information more easily	*"In a FtF session you say a lot, but afterwards patients also forget quickly. Now they can review what they've learned as many times as they want."* (T10, experience)
	(+) reducing travel time	*"In other countries, factors such as distances and climate play a role, but of course in the middle of the country we have traffic jams. bCBT is very nice for this."* (T9, experience)
	(+) more contact with patient	*"Throughout the treatment you have more frequent short contact moments, which are actually very good."* (T10, experience)
	(+) sharing content with system	*"For the patient you remove the treatment from therapist's office to their own home."* (T12, no/little experience).
	(+) effect of writing	*"Patients have to write, this is for many a very good instrument to order things and gain new insights. I find the writing a very positive addition to the verbal component."* (T15, experience)
	(+) monitoring homework	*"I find it very attractive that there is more control over the homework that they have or haven't done."* (T2, experience)
	(+) facilitating patient self-efficacy	*"In the online part a degree of independence makes patients themselves engage with the treatment. I think that they attribute treatment success to themselves, more than with FtF treatment."* (T22, experience)
Negative effects	(−) no gain in time, costs more	*"I find it takes more time than I expected. Especially if you're still unfamiliar with the module."* (T7, no/little experience)
	(−) unsuitable content	*"I had a traumatized patient, because she couldn't have children. The first example on the platform was 'I have children and I want to be a good mother...'."* (T27, no/little experience)
Treatment format	(−/+) discussion on structure protocol	*"I find it difficult to be flexible in the protocol and not to become a sort of CBT machine."* (T21, no/little experience)
	(−/+) discussion on freedom in protocol to explore depression	*"Usually, when I start without the platform, I think 'never mind'. But also, when the patient isn't ready for it initially, you can say 'Later on, we will start with the online platform'."* (T31, no/little experience)
	(−/+) discussion on 'what is blended'	*"I don't think it's 50/50. The main focus is more on the FtF sessions. I notice that the conversations and the modules do not always run parallel to each other."* (T14, no/little experience)

Table 5. *Cont.*

Subtheme	Influencing Factors	Illustrative Quotes
	(−/+) discussion on introduction platform	*"Whether you start treatment with an online module, right at the outset or only when a basis has been formed, is dependent on the therapist. I think am very comfortable with starting right away."* (T1, no/little experience)
Therapeutic relationship	(−/+) discussion on quality therapeutic relationship	*"It's possible to build a therapeutic relationship, but sometimes it isn't. Yet I think that this isn't dependent on bCBT. Also, with FtF therapy it's possible to succeed in building a therapeutic relationship and sometimes not."* (T15, experience)
Online feedback skills	(−) time providing feedback (−) permanent character of online feedback	*"I reflect more on what I want to write, that is perhaps the reason why it takes more time."* (T7, no/little experience) *"It's difficult to assess whether someone has understood something in the way you intended. If this happens in FtF contact you can talk around it, look friendly and explain. In black and white this is not possible."* (T5, no/little experience)
	(+) connection online feedback and FtF conversations	*"I notice that patients like to come back to a point during the conversations, to go through the exercises together."* (T12, no/little experience)
Dropout & safety	(−/+) discussion on safety risks	*"In the meantime, I experienced that it's okay if the patient also comes to the FtF sessions. You've to make this clear at the start. The risk you lose contact is lower than I expected."* (T9, experience)
	(+) bCBT has no extra risks with regards to suicidal ideation	*"I thought that if you see someone less that it'd be more difficult to assess the suicide risk. But it can just as well lower the threshold to say something online more easily than to discuss FtF."* (T31, no/little experience)
	(+) drop-out bCBT = drop-out CBT	*"I don't have one type of patient that drops out of blended. It's very unpredictable who completes it."* (T30, experience)
	(+) sufficient patient data safety	*"I understood that the online platform is very safe, safer than email."* (T33, experience)

Note. (−) factor that influenced the bCBT uptake negatively, (+) factor that influenced the bCBT uptake positively, (−/+) factor that influenced the bCBT uptake positively and negatively.

Effectiveness for Depression

Therapists agreed that bCBT offered a good foundation for treating patients with depression. Nevertheless, they also found that the therapeutic content of the online sessions needed improvement, especially for patients with severe depressive symptoms who were characterized by more inactivity, complex problems, and longer treatment history. Whether 'the blended' treatment format exists, remained a question. Not based on research findings, but based on their experience, therapists uniformly thought that bCBT and FtF CBT could be equally effective. bCBT mainly helped to structure treatment and both patient and therapist to remain focused.

Positive Effects

The most cited positive effect was containing therapist drift; platform functionalities facilitated therapist (and patient) focus and protocol adherence more than in regular CBT because of the pre-set structure of bCBT. Therapists found it easier to control homework assignments and patients knew what was scheduled next. It was believed that all this positively impacted the quality of the treatment. An additional effect was that other diagnoses besides depression (e.g., autism) or certain problems (e.g., suicidal ideation, non-adherence, low cognitive capacities) were made more visible to the therapists at an earlier treatment stage. This was due to a discrepancy between online symptom monitoring, patients' online expressions, and what was said and shown in FtF sessions. Plus, for therapists, it was more noticeable from the patients' writing skills what the cognitive abilities were.

In the therapists' experience, patients found it easier to remember what was discussed in FtF sessions with bCBT. The information on the platform supported therapists—they had more information available, not only about depression but on other treatment options as well (e.g., sleep, self-image). In addition, because patients with depression often have concentration problems, the unlimited and easy access to treatment information and psychoeducation was very useful.

Reducing travel-time was mentioned as being very convenient for patients, not only for practical reasons (e.g., having children, employment), but also for therapists. bCBT provided an extra tool to stay connected with patients, especially in cases of no-show. Therapists discovered that patients shared the platform content with their immediate circle more easily (e.g., partner, family, or friends). Plus, the effect of writing on the online platform was a big advantage to patients. Patients wrote down their problems, came to new insights, and shared shameful problems more easily because of the distance effect and having time for reflection. bCBT offered patients greater responsibility. As for self-efficacy, some therapists thought that patients tended to attribute the treatment success to themselves more than in FtF treatment.

Negative Effects

Most therapists questioned whether bCBT could shorten treatments and solve waiting list problems. First, therapists spent a lot of time getting to know the platform and secondly, providing therapy via the online environment was time-consuming in contrast to expectations. Perhaps it might be timesaving in the future. However, the common thought was that bCBT is 'just another way of doing the same thing'. Some felt that there is a long way to go before blended interventions are considered equally effective as regular CBT by therapists in general.

Some judged the content on the platform to be too textual, too complex, or too superficial, thus requiring repeat sessions and extra clarification. Moreover, sometimes patients did not recognize themselves in the text and video examples; some found the content pejorative, overly directive, or too intense, resulting in drop-out or even worsening of their mood. Therefore, some therapists felt a strong need for personalization of the content to adapt to the patients' preferences and background.

Treatment Format

While experienced therapists unanimously stated that the pre-set structure of the blended protocol was very beneficial, for therapists with less experience, this was not the case. For them, the protocol was too structured and therefore inflexible. Experienced therapists, who had a better overview of all the functionalities, mentioned that bCBT was very similar to FtF CBT, in which you also adapt to the protocol when needed.

Therapists had different views on the ratio of FtF versus online sessions within bCBT. Some regarded and used bCBT as an addition to the regular number of FtF sessions. Moreover, for some the question 'what is blended?' remained. Therapists had different views on degrees of 'blendedness'. Repeatedly, it was seen as an interchange of FtF sessions with the functionalities of the online platform. For some patients 50%–50% was considered beneficial, for others 90% FtF and 10% online was more appropriate.

Another issue was the time point at which the online platform was introduced. Some therapists preferred to start with weekly FtF sessions and introduced the platform at a later date. For them, it felt unnatural and too distracting for patients to meet every two weeks instead of weekly in the first phase of treatment. They wanted more time to establish a foundation, especially for patients who lacked insight into their depression. Other therapists, who thought it would be better to start with the online platform at once, reasoned that the threshold (for patients and therapists) may be higher when the platform is introduced at a later stage. These therapists also imagined that it motivated patients to be focused from the beginning with the support of the platform.

Therapeutic Relationship

Regarding the quality of a therapeutic relationship in bCBT, therapists' opinions were divided. In the beginning, some doubted whether it was possible to develop a therapeutic relationship because they would see patients less FtF, but changed their opinion later on. In some therapists' experience, it was challenging to build a therapeutic relationship compared to regular CBT; when a patient experienced difficulties with the online platform and asked more attention from the therapist, this frustrated the contact because it was at the expense of the time they had FtF. Nevertheless, others experienced that the relationship in bCBT was similar or even better compared to FtF treatment. bCBT reinforced the relationship, since there was more frequent contact throughout. In addition, the treatment course was more visible to therapists because of online monitoring and this also positively influenced the relationship. Importantly, as in every treatment, the relationship was mainly perceived as more dependent on patient motivation and activation than other factors such as online contact.

Online Feedback Skills

Therapists agreed that every therapist is able to provide online feedback. However, learning how to provide feedback took time and for many, felt like 'a job in its own right'. They were needed for tips, tools, and examples; how to address something negative, how to handle or prevent miscommunication, how to write in a concise manner, how to make feedback personalized and adapt to different patient types. In contrast to FtF sessions, where therapists are able to correct themselves, everything that is written online, has a permanent character: for some, online feedback thus felt uncomfortable.

Therapists stressed the importance of connecting to the language of the patient. They found they had to be careful not to use difficult terminology or be too distant in their language. Most of all, they had to plan sufficient time to write feedback. Therapists noticed that writing online feedback became faster with more experience. Connecting online feedback and topics in FtF sessions and vice versa, was experienced as helpful and was done quite frequently.

Drop-Out and Safety

Two safety risks cited predominantly by inexperienced therapists were the suggestion of 24/7 accessibility to patients and not being able to see how patients reacted to therapist feedback or other online information. Experienced therapists did not mention this or had learned that this was not an issue.

Regarding a much-discussed risk of suicidal ideation, therapists experienced that when there was a clear agreement with patients on not expressing crisis situations on the platform, bCBT had no extra risks compared to FtF treatment. Importantly, it even gave therapists more rapid awareness of whether patients were losing contact. In addition, bCBT provided therapists with an extra preventive communication tool.

Furthermore, experienced therapists reported that there was no specific type of patient that dropped out. Sometimes therapists saw patients who started enthusiastically, but dropped out easily. Importantly, they thought this was no different than with regular CBT: patients dropped out because of certain patient characteristics or other problems than for bCBT-related issues.

Overall, therapists expressed that safety of patient data on the online platform is guaranteed sufficiently. Sharing patient data with, for example, a helpdesk, is still something that therapists were reluctant to do and prevented them from contacting the helpdesk when technical issues occurred. They often then tried to solve their issues with colleagues, but often also broke off the online sessions. Some patients seemed too lax when it came to their data safety, and some were distrustful. Therapists emphasized that it is their responsibility to explain how safe the online platform is, but that this was not clear to all therapists.

4. Discussion

In this study, therapists expressed overall satisfaction with providing bCBT to patients with depression. The perceived usability of the online platform was sufficient. This was also found by other studies exploring patients' perspectives on usability and satisfaction [21,36]. This study showed that therapists see room for improvement with regard to platform usability (e.g., lack of integration with other administrative systems), therapists' work routines, and guideline use on bCBT. From interviews in this study, it became clear that there are specific barriers that prevented therapists from providing bCBT to patients with depression, such as a lack of ongoing support for technical and clinical issues with bCBT. In addition, therapists reported several practical and therapeutic challenges in routine care such as not experiencing timesaving. Nevertheless, there have been factors that might have influenced the uptake positively as well.

4.1. Barriers to bCBT Uptake

Less experienced bCBT therapists felt several barriers prevented them from providing bCBT. First, they found that the training was not sufficient to enable them to adopt bCBT into their work routine. This was partly because the training mainly covered technical aspects and did not provide sufficient guidance on how to work in a blended way with the protocol and how to communicate online. In addition, after undergoing training, ongoing support and attention for bCBT was limited or absent. This was also a reported therapist barrier by Folker et al. [37] who identified implementation challenges perceived by therapists and managers of iCBT in routine care settings in five European countries. Moreover, inexperienced therapists were unsure about the indication for bCBT and the eligibility of the patients. A third issue was that some therapists experienced low patient demand for bCBT. A fourth hindering factor was that for a number of the therapists, the added value of bCBT in terms of clinical effectiveness remained unclear; for others, fear (e.g., of doing something wrong) or distrust (e.g., regarding the intentions of health insurance companies) stood in the way of considering bCBT.

4.2. Challenges with bCBT

Once therapists started working with bCBT, they experienced several challenges. They had difficulty integrating bCBT into their daily workflow. Not only because of technical disconnections with existing IT-systems for patients' administration, but also because of uncertainties regarding the bCBT protocol and logistic integration into their daily therapeutic and administrative schedules. Besides, therapists lacked the conviction that bCBT saved time; for some, it even generated a higher workload, especially in the beginning, and providing online feedback is considered time-consuming as well. It can be estimated, that on average per feedback message, 30 min of therapist time is needed [13]. Internal helpdesks were unable to support therapists sufficiently which even discouraged some from further providing bCBT.

Moreover, therapists displayed different interpretations of the protocol which partly resulted for some in using the online platform on top of the FtF treatment instead of replacing a portion of the FtF sessions. This was previously reported in a naturalistic study on bCBT uptake in routine care as well [38], making the implementation more costly than intended. Kenter et al. [38] argued that their therapists may have needed more extensive training to master specific bCBT skills (e.g., providing online feedback) and that clear guidelines on how to use bCBT in routine practice by the MHO would have helped the therapist to provide bCBT more efficiently. Plus, using the online platform on top of the FtF treatment may result in patient dissatisfaction. A study on patients' experiences with bCBT showed that a diminished interplay between the online and FtF sessions was unsatisfactory for patients, as therapists were less aware of patient activity on the online platform and limited time was made available to discuss the online activity in the FtF sessions [39].

4.3. Advantages of bCBT

One of the main reported advantages of bCBT was the focus and pre-set structure that made therapists and their patients more adherent to the protocol and contained therapist drift. This was also experienced by several therapists who worked with bCBT [14,19] or blended group therapy [40] for depression. Although content improvement (e.g., online patient examples) for severely depressed patients was considered necessary, therapists agreed that bCBT is a good treatment format for the (complex) patient group therapists see in daily practice. They found that bCBT was in many ways similar to FtF CBT when it comes to patient eligibility, effectiveness, therapeutic relationship, and drop-out: 'it is CBT in another format'. Many believed that the implementation phase is still in its infancy; it might be a long way to go before all therapists accept blended interventions as being equally effective to FtF therapy. This idea is also partly justified since the first studies on clinical effects on blended interventions show that it is at least as effective [12,13]. Nonetheless, it is thought that bCBT will eventually be included in care pathways in the future because of the perceived benefits for patients and therapists (e.g., pre-set structure, number of flexible contact moments on demand, information access); an important precondition is to continue to be combined with FtF contact, as providing stand-alone guided iCBT might not yet be realistic for most therapists in routine practice, where FtF treatment is the norm.

4.4. Level of Experience

In our study, therapists with bCBT experience reported different views on safety, flexibility and personalization of the protocol, patient eligibility, and therapeutic relationship than therapists who lacked experience. For example, non-experienced therapists assumed that there were many reasons why patients would be ineligible for bCBT, such as severe depressive symptoms, or found this difficult to assess. By contrast, more experienced therapists stated that it was impossible to predict eligibility; in principle, any patient could be offered bCBT. This may indicate that with experience, perceptions on these important clinical factors of bCBT will change and that when promoting uptake, therapists' needs can shift. This is consistent with Feijt et al. [41] who showed that there are different barriers and facilitators depending on the level of therapist experience with online services, and that potentially, the experience level has unique requirements to be addressed when it comes to the uptake of Internet-based interventions.

4.5. Limitations and Strengths

Although some therapists in this study were skeptical about the effectiveness of bCBT or had negative experiences, all were quite open-minded toward bCBT. Selection bias in our sample is possible, as untrained therapists or those not interested in participating in the study were not reached and therapists were identified through their team managers, and other specially appointed members of different teams. This could have diminished the positive view on bCBT.

Another point is the limited transferability of our findings to other national contexts. In the Netherlands, the digital infrastructure is quite good and MHO's and therapists have the experience that every patient has proper equipment. Moreover, bCBT is covered by health care insurance companies in the same way as face-to-face CBT. Compared to other countries, the Netherlands and others, including Sweden and the United Kingdom, can be considered a frontrunner in implementing bCBT within routine practice [16]. On the other hand, our findings can be taken into account by the 'followers' in the earlier stages of developing, testing, and implementing bCBT.

A strength of this study is the usage of data triangulation to record the perspective of a diverse group of therapists, with different professional backgrounds, differences in experiences with bCBT for depression, and exposure to various implementation strategies from a number of mental health care organizations.

4.6. Future Uptake of bCBT

To speed up bCBT uptake, it is important to identify how barriers can be overcome, challenges solved, and how successes in routine care can be strengthened. From the field of implementation research, it is known that implementation strategies for innovations in mental health care need 'to address multiple levels and barriers to change, (and) are interwoven and packaged as a protocolized or branded implementation intervention' [42]. Based on this and on the findings of this study, the following strategies can be considered in practice and in research to move forward in the implementation of bCBT:

1. Dissemination strategies: to change the focus of cost-effectiveness of bCBT towards personalization, adherence, and treatment quality improvement in disseminating information to therapists and patients. Within organizations, the uptake might gain from informing and motivating therapists and subsequently patients as well. There is a lot of room for improvement when it comes to sufficient knowledge about bCBT. Outside the organizations, patient demand can be stimulated by general practitioners and health insurance companies. Further, although evidence-based knowledge on bCBT is slowly becoming more available, this should be more widespread among patients, therapists, MHOs, and health insurance companies.
2. Top down strategies: bCBT must be embedded top-down from start to finish overcoming its mere project status in many of the MHOs. This could be achieved by intensifying and extending training beyond technical aspects, and by facilitating the integration of ongoing support into existing consultation structures, (instead of creating special consultation options), in order to exchange knowledge and experience with bCBT. It would also help to remind therapists to offer bCBT to patients and to solve technical disconnections with administration- and other IT-systems within a well-equipped help desk. Whether imposing minimum usage norms (e.g., that 25% of the treatments must be blended in the Netherlands) could have a promoting effect is unclear, as this causes resistance for some, but motivated others.
3. Bottom-up strategies: Fragmented use and individual uptake of the blended protocol can create a risk of it being costlier and of leading to a protocolled manner of working. Therapists' need

to personalize modules might be a result of uncertainty and their limited knowledge of all functionalities within the module and platform. Thus, besides a top-down approach, therapists might be more motivated and skilled if uptake is stimulated on a bottom-up basis, through discussing it on the work floor: For instance, it could help to start implementation with a small rollout with a motivated team of therapists, focusing on content development, enhancing online feedback skills and protocol use; to let the therapists be (co-) creators of modules; to construct a place and time within MHOs where therapists can think of ways to further develop bCBT; to experiment; to keep lines with the technical innovations on the platform within reach; including recurring evaluation in order to adapt strategies on the level of therapist experience and updates of the platform.

4.7. Future Research

Testing strategies for uptake would be a fruitful area for further research. The European project, ImpleMentAll (www.implementall.eu), will hopefully provide routine practice with more knowledge as this is uncharted territory for Internet interventions in mental health care [43]. In ImpleMentAll, personalized implementation strategies will be tested to facilitate the use of Internet-based and blended interventions in routine care in several different countries.

In addition, it would support uptake of bCBT to further investigate the ratio and integration of online and FtF sessions. So far, research has focused on an equal distribution. However, it is reasonable to think that depending on the severity of the symptoms, the proportion of blended could be adapted. Moreover, it would be interesting for future studies to also look at the patient perspectives on blended care, preferably done using dyad interviews with their therapists to generate a rich, deeper understanding of the relevant factors in bCBT uptake.

5. Conclusions

Overall, the therapists in this study were satisfied with providing bCBT to patients with depression. That said, a large group of therapists is still wondering how much FtF contact should be included in blended. Plus, important preconditions for implementation were unmet and the technical infrastructure is not free from teething problems. It cannot be expected from therapists that uptake happens spontaneously. It can be considered positive that having bCBT experience can be a possible key to change a therapist's view on important factors such as eligibility and drop-out. Therapists found that there is a good base that can be further developed in terms of ongoing technical support, therapeutic support from their peers and supervisors, while at the same time strategically implementing bCBT on an organizational level to facilitate therapists in the transition of integrating bCBT into their daily practice.

Supplementary Materials: The following are available online at http://www.mdpi.com/2077-0383/9/1/91/s1, File S1: Topic list focus groups, File S2: Topic list semi-structured interviews experienced therapists, File S3: Topic list semi-structured interviews non-experienced therapists.

Author Contributions: All authors have contributed substantially to the work reported. All authors critically revised the paper. Conceptualization, M.M., E.D., D.J.F.v.S., H.R. and J.H.S.; Data curation, M.M.; Formal analysis, M.M., C.v.G. and S.D.; Funding acquisition, H.R. and J.H.S.; Investigation, M.M., C.v.G. and S.D.; Methodology, M.M., E.D., D.J.F.v.S., S.D., H.R. and J.H.S.; Software, M.M.; Supervision, H.R. and J.H.S.; Validation, M.M., C.v.G. and S.D.; Visualization, M.M.; Writing—original draft, M.M.; Writing—review & editing, M.M., C.v.G., E.D., D.J.F.v.S., S.D., H.R. and J.H.S. All authors have read and agreed to the published version of the manuscript.

Funding: This research was partially funded under the Information and Communications Technologies (ICT) Policy Support Programme as part of the Competitiveness and Innovation Framework Programme (CIP) by the European Community, grant number 621000.

Acknowledgments: The authors would like to thank several people for their contributions: Thuur Smet (data extraction), Nanda Mooij, Bep Verkerk (data management), Martine de Meijer (transcribing interviews). We also would like to thank the therapists and the participating mental health care organizations for their time and effort.

Conflicts of Interest: The authors declare no conflict of interest. The funders had no role in the design of the study; in the collection, analyses, or interpretation of data; in the writing of the manuscript, or in the decision to publish the results. The authors were not involved in the development of the bCBT module.

References

1. Cuijpers, P.; Noma, H.; Karyotaki, E.; Cipriani, A.; Furukawa, T.A. Effectiveness and Acceptability of Cognitive Behavior Therapy Delivery Formats in Adults with Depression: A Network Meta-analysis. *JAMA Psychiatry* **2019**, *76*, 700–707. [CrossRef] [PubMed]
2. National Institute for Clinical Excellence. Depression: The treatment and management of depression in adults. In *Clinical Guideline 90*; NICE: London, UK, 2009.
3. World Health Organization. Depression and Other Common Mental Disorders: Global Health Estimates. In *World Health Organization Report*; World Health Organization: Geneva, Switzerland, 2017; pp. 1–24.
4. Boerema, A.M.; Kleiboer, A.; Beekman, A.T.F.; van Zoonen, K.; Dijkshoorn, H.; Cuijpers, P. Determinants of help-seeking behavior in depression: A cross-sectional study. *BMC Psychiatry* **2016**, *16*. [CrossRef] [PubMed]
5. Andrews, G.; Basu, A.; Cuijpers, P.; Craske, M.G.; McEvoy, P.; English, C.L.; Newby, J.M. Computer therapy for the anxiety and depression disorders is effective, acceptable and practical health care: An updated meta-analysis. *J. Anxiety Disord.* **2018**, *55*, 70–78. [CrossRef] [PubMed]
6. Karyotaki, E.; Riper, H.; Twisk, J.; Hoogendoorn, A.; Kleiboer, A.; Mira, A.; MacKinnon, A.; Meyer, B.; Botella, C.; Littlewood, E.; et al. Efficacy of self-guided internet-based cognitive behavioral therapy in the treatment of depressive symptoms a meta-analysis of individual participant data. *JAMA Psychiatry* **2017**, *74*, 351–359. [CrossRef] [PubMed]
7. Titov, N.; Dear, B.; Nielssen, O.; Staples, L.; Hadjistavropoulos, H.; Nugent, M.; Adlam, K.; Nordgreen, T.; Bruvik, K.H.; Hovland, A.; et al. ICBT in routine care: A descriptive analysis of successful clinics in five countries. *Internet Interv.* **2018**, *13*, 108–115. [CrossRef]
8. Erbe, D.; Psych, D.; Eichert, H.C.; Riper, H.; Ebert, D.D. Blending face-to-face and internet-based interventions for the treatment of mental disorders in adults: Systematic review. *J. Med. Internet Res.* **2017**, *19*. [CrossRef]
9. Hadjistavropoulos, H.D.; Nugent, M.M.; Dirkse, D.; Pugh, N. Implementation of internet-delivered cognitive behavior therapy within community mental health clinics: A process evaluation using the consolidated framework for implementation research. *BMC Psychiatry* **2017**, *17*. [CrossRef]
10. Definition Blended Treatment Heleen Riper. Triple-E Website. Available online: https://www.triple-ehealth.nl/en/projects-cat/depressie/ and http://www.webcitation.org/6wZFBY9pX (accessed on 18 January 2018).
11. Kleiboer, A.; Smit, J.; Bosmans, J.; Ruwaard, J.; Andersson, G.; Topooco, N.; Berger, T.; Krieger, T.; Botella, C.; Baños, R.; et al. European COMPARative Effectiveness research on blended Depression treatment versus treatment-as-usual (E-COMPARED): Study protocol for a randomized controlled, non-inferiority trial in eight European countries. *Trials* **2016**, *17*. [CrossRef]
12. Romijn, G.; Batelaan, N.; Koning, J.; van Balkom, A.; de Leeuw, A.; Benning, F.; Hakkaart-van Roijen, L.; Riper, H. Effectiveness and cost-effectiveness of blended cognitive-behavioural therapy for anxiety disorders in specialised mental health care: A 15-week randomised controlled trial with 1-year follow-up. 2019; accepted.
13. Kooistra, L.C.; Wiersma, J.E.; Ruwaard, J.J.; Neijenhuijs, K.; Lokkerbol, J.; Smit, F.; van Oppen, P.; Riper, H. Costs and effectiveness of blended versus standard cognitive behavioral therapy for depressed outpatients in routine specialized mental healthcare: A pilot randomized controlled trial. *J. Med. Internet Res.* **2019**, *21*. [CrossRef]
14. Mansson, K.N.; Skagius Ruiz, E.; Gervind, E.; Dahlin, M.; Andersson, G. Development and initial evaluation of an Internet-based support system for face-to-face cognitive behavior therapy: A proof of concept study. *J. Med. Internet Res.* **2013**, *15*, e280. [CrossRef] [PubMed]
15. Thase, M.E.; Wright, J.H.; Eells, T.D.; Barrett, M.S.; Wisniewski, S.R.; Balasubramani, G.K.; McCrone, P.; Brown, G.K. Improving the Efficiency of Psychotherapy for Depression: Computer-Assisted Versus Standard CBT. *Am. J. Psychiatry* **2017**, *175*. [CrossRef] [PubMed]
16. Topooco, N.; Riper, H.; Araya, R.; Berking, M.; Brunn, M.; Chevreul, K.; Cieslak, R.; Ebert, D.D.; Etchmendy, E.; Herrero, R.; et al. Attitudes towards digital treatment for depression: A European stakeholder survey. *Internet Interv.* **2017**, *8*, 1–9. [CrossRef]
17. Vis, C.; Kleiboer, A.; Prior, R.; Bønes, E.; Cavallo, M.; Clark, S.A.; Dozeman, E.; Ebert, D.; Etzelmueller, A.; Favaretto, G.; et al. Implementing and up-scaling evidence-based eMental health in Europe: The study protocol for the MasterMind project. *Internet Interv.* **2015**, *2*. [CrossRef]

18. Mol, M.; Dozeman, E.; van Schaik, D.J.F.; Vis, C.P.C.D.; Riper, H.; Smit, J.H. The therapist's role in the implementation of internet-based cognitive behavioural therapy for patients with depression: Study protocol. *BMC Psychiatry* **2016**, *16*, 338. [CrossRef]
19. Titzler, I.; Saruhanjan, K.; Berking, M.; Riper, H.; Ebert, D.D. Barriers and facilitators for the implementation of blended psychotherapy for depression: A qualitative pilot study of therapists' perspective. *Internet Interv.* **2018**, *12*, 150–164. [CrossRef]
20. Denzin, N.K. Triangulation 2.0 *. *J. Mix. Methods Res.* **2012**, *6*, 80–88. [CrossRef]
21. Kooistra, L.C.; Ruwaard, J.; Wiersma, J.E.; van Oppen, P.; van der Vaart, R.; van Gemert-Pijnen, J.E.W.C.; Riper, H. Development and initial evaluation of blended cognitive behavioural treatment for major depression in routine specialized mental health care. *Internet Interv.* **2016**, *4*, 61–71. [CrossRef]
22. Regulation (EU) 2016/679 of the European Parliament and of the Council of 27 April 2016 on the Protection of Natural Persons with Regard to the Processing of Personal Data and on the Free Movement of Such Data, and Repealing Directive 95/46/EC (General Data Protection Regulation). Official Journal of the European Union L 119/1. Available online: http://data.europa.eu/eli/reg/2016/679/oj (accessed on 10 December 2019).
23. Brooke, J. SUS-A quick and dirty usability scale. *Usability Eval. Ind.* **1996**, *189*, 4–7.
24. Mol, M.; van Schaik, A.; Dozeman, E.; Ruwaard, J.; Vis, C.; Ebert, D.D.; Etzelmueller, A.; Mathiasen, K.; Moles, B.; Mora, T.; et al. Dimensionality of System Usability Scale among professionals using internet-based interventions for depression: A confirmatory factor analysis. 2019; accepted.
25. Sauro, J. *A Practical Guide to the System Usability Scale: Background, Benchmarks & Best Practices*; Measuring Usability LLC: Denver, CO, USA, 2011.
26. Sauro, J.; Lewis, J.R. Quantifying user research. In *Quantifying the User Experience*; Elsevier: Amsterdam, The Netherlands, 2016; pp. 9–18. [CrossRef]
27. Attkisson, C.C.; Greenfield, T.K. *The Client Satisfaction Questionnaire (CSQ) Scales. Outcome Assessment in Clinical Practice*; Williams & Wilkins: Baltimore, MD, USA, 1995.
28. Boß, L.; Lehr, D.; Reis, D.; Vis, C.; Riper, H.; Berking, M.; Ebert, D.D. Reliability and validity of assessing user satisfaction with web-based health interventions. *J. Med. Internet Res.* **2016**, *18*, e234. [CrossRef]
29. Glasgow, R.E.; Vogt, T.M.; Boles, S.M. Evaluating the public health impact of health promotion interventions: The RE-AIM framework. *Am. J. Public Health* **1999**, *89*, 1322–1327. [CrossRef]
30. Kidholm, K.; Ekeland, A.G.; Jensen, L.K.; Rasmussen, J.; Pedersen, C.D.; Bowes, A.; Flottorp, S.A.; Bech, M. A model for assessment of telemedicine applications: Mast. *Int. J. Technol. Assess. Health Care* **2012**, *28*, 44–51. [CrossRef] [PubMed]
31. May, C.R.; Mair, F.; Finch, T.; MacFarlane, A.; Dowrick, C.; Treweek, S.; Rapley, T.; Ballini, L.; Ong, B.N.; Rogers, A.; et al. Development of a theory of implementation and integration: Normalization Process Theory. *Implement. Sci.* **2009**, *4*. [CrossRef] [PubMed]
32. Kivi, M.; Eriksson, M.C.M.; Hange, D.; Petersson, E.L.; Björkelund, C.; Johansson, B. Experiences and attitudes of primary care therapists in the implementation and use of internet-based treatment in Swedish primary care settings. *Internet Interv.* **2015**, *2*, 248–256. [CrossRef]
33. Wilhelmsen, M.; Hoifodt, R.S.; Kolstrup, N.; Waterloo, K.; Eisemann, M.; Chenhall, R.; Risor, M.B. Norwegian general practitioners' perspectives on implementation of a guided web-based cognitive behavioral therapy for depression: A qualitative study. *J. Med. Internet Res.* **2014**, *16*, e208. [CrossRef]
34. Braun, V.; Clarke, V. Using thematic analysis in psychology. *Qual. Res. Psychol.* **2006**, *3*, 77–101. [CrossRef]
35. Fleiss, L.; Levin, B.; Paik, M.C. The measurement of interrater agreement. In *Statistical Methods for Rates and Proportions*, 3rd ed.; John Wiley & Sons, Inc.: Hoboken, NJ, USA, 2003.
36. Etzelmueller, A.; Radkovsky, A.; Hannig, W.; Berking, M.; Ebert, D.D. Patient's experience with blended video- and internet based cognitive behavioural therapy service in routine care. *Internet Interv.* **2018**, *12*, 165–175. [CrossRef]
37. Folker, A.P.; Mathiasen, K.; Lauridsen, S.M.; Stenderup, E.; Dozeman, E.; Folker, M.P. Implementing internet-delivered cognitive behavior therapy for common mental health disorders: A comparative case study of implementation challenges perceived by therapists and managers in five European internet services. *Internet Interv.* **2018**, *11*, 60–70. [CrossRef]
38. Kenter, R.M.F.; van de Ven, P.M.; Cuijpers, P.; Koole, G.; Niamat, S.; Gerrits, R.S.; Willems, M.; van Straten, A. Costs and effects of Internet cognitive behavioral treatment blended with face-to-face treatment: Results from a naturalistic study. *Internet Interv.* **2015**, *2*, 77–83. [CrossRef]

39. Urech, A.; Krieger, T.; Möseneder, L.; Biaggi, A.; Vincent, A.; Poppe, C.; Meyer, B.; Riper, H.; Berger, T. A patient post hoc perspective on advantages and disadvantages of blended cognitive behaviour therapy for depression: A qualitative content analysis. *Psychother. Res.* **2018**, *29*, 986–998. [CrossRef]
40. Schuster, R.; Sigl, S.; Berger, T.; Laireiter, A.R. Patients' Experiences of Web- and Mobile-Assisted Group Therapy for Depression and Implications of the Group Setting: Qualitative Follow-Up Study. *JMIR Ment. Health* **2018**, *5*, e49. [CrossRef] [PubMed]
41. Feijt, M.A.; De Kort, Y.A.W.; Bongers, I.M.B.; IJsselsteijn, W.A. Perceived drivers and barriers to the adoption of eMental health by psychologists: The construction of the levels of adoption of eMental health model. *J. Med. Internet Res.* **2018**, *20*. [CrossRef] [PubMed]
42. Powell, B.J.; McMillen, J.C.; Proctor, E.K.; Carpenter, C.R.; Griffey, R.T.; Bunger, A.C.; Glass, J.E.; York, J.L. A compilation of strategies for implementing clinical innovations in health and mental health. *Med. Care Res. Rev.* **2012**, *69*, 123–157. [CrossRef] [PubMed]
43. Bührmann, L.; Schuurmans, J.; Ruwaard, J. Tailored Implementation of Internet-based Cognitive Behavioural Therapy in the Multinational Context of the ImpleMentAll Project: A Study Protocol for a Stepped Wedge Cluster Randomized Trial. under review.

Journal of
Clinical Medicine

Article

Working Alliance in Blended Versus Face-to-Face Cognitive Behavioral Treatment for Patients with Depression in Specialized Mental Health Care

Lisa Kooistra [1,2,*], Jeroen Ruwaard [2,3,†], Jenneke Wiersma [2], Patricia van Oppen [2,3] and Heleen Riper [1,2,3]

1 Department of Clinical, Neuro-and Developmental Psychology and the Amsterdam Public Health Research Institute, Vrije Universiteit Amsterdam, van der Boechorststraat 7, 1081 BT Amsterdam, The Netherlands; m.m.riper@vu.nl

2 Department of Research and Innovation, GGZ inGeest Specialized Mental Health Care, Oldenaller 1, 1081 HJ Amsterdam, The Netherlands; jennekewiersma@gmail.com (J.W.); p.vanoppen@ggzingeest.nl (P.v.O.)

3 Department of Psychiatry and the Amsterdam Public Health Research Institute, GGZ inGeest/Amsterdam UMC, Vrije Universiteit, de Boelelaan 1117, 1081 HV Amsterdam, The Netherlands

* Correspondence: l.kooistra@ggzingeest.nl

† Died July 2019.

Received: 30 November 2019; Accepted: 18 January 2020; Published: 27 January 2020

Abstract: This study investigates working alliance in blended cognitive behavioral therapy (bCBT) for depressed adults in specialized mental health care. Patients were randomly allocated to bCBT ($n = 47$) or face-to-face CBT ($n = 45$). After 10 weeks of treatment, both patients and therapists in the two groups rated the therapeutic alliance on the Working Alliance Inventory Short-Form Revised (WAI-SR; Task, Bond, Goal, and composite scores). No between-group differences were found in relation to either patient or therapist alliance ratings, which were high in both groups. In the full sample, a moderate positive association was found between patient and therapist ratings on Task ($\varrho = 0.41$, 95% CI 0.20; 0.59), but no significant associations emerged on other components or composite scores. At 30 weeks, within-and between-group associations between alliance and changes in depression severity (QIDS, Quick Inventory of Depressive Symptomatology) were analyzed with linear mixed models. The analyses revealed an association between depression over time, patient-rated alliance, and group ($p < 0.001$). In face-to-face CBT, but not in bCBT, lower depression scores were associated with higher alliance ratings. The online component in bCBT may have led patients to evaluate the working alliance differently from patients receiving face-to-face CBT only.

Keywords: major depressive disorder; blended cognitive behavioral treatment; specialized mental health care; working alliance; randomized controlled trial

1. Introduction

Although major depressive disorder (MDD) is a common and severely disabling illness [1], many individuals with MDD have limited access to mental health care and trained therapists [2–4]. This has prompted development of interventions requiring less therapist involvement, such as self-help interventions [5,6], and online psychotherapy [7,8]. Various studies have shown that online interventions, most often based on cognitive behavioral therapy, are effective in treating common mental disorders [9–13]—especially when patients receive professional guidance, for example, via secured e-mail exchange or an online treatment platform [5,9,14,15]. The past few years have seen growing interest in hybrid treatment approaches, which either combine or integrate face-to-face and online therapy [16]. As this is a relatively new form of treatment, evidence on effectiveness is still scarce. Initial evaluations suggest that blended treatment can be effective in decreasing depression severity [17–24].

The consequent modifications in the amounts and forms of contact between therapists and patients in online and blended interventions, as compared with face-to-face treatments, have led some therapists to worry that therapeutic alliance might be negatively impacted [18] and that this could weaken treatment outcomes. This is relevant, as therapeutic alliance is considered an important common factor in psychotherapy [25]. A stronger alliance between therapists and patients has been shown to be moderately associated with better treatment outcomes in face-to-face treatment [26–28], with meta-analyses reporting overall weighted averages of $r = 0.28$ (95% CI 0.26; 0.30) in psychotherapy for mental disorders [28] and $r = 0.26$ (95% CI 0.19; 0.32) in cognitive behavioral therapy (CBT) for depression [29]. However, such associations might be moderated by other factors. For example, assessment of alliance in a later phase of treatment may detect stronger associations between alliance and treatment effect than early assessment [28,29], and the alliance–outcome association has been found weaker for therapist-rated alliance than patient-rated alliance [29]. Associations might also be positively impacted if patient and therapist ratings of working alliance more strongly concur [30], or if patients have had fewer prior depressive episodes [31].

For blended depression treatments, available evidence on therapeutic alliance is still limited. Initial evaluations showed patient-rated alliance in online interventions to be high and comparable to ratings in face-to-face treatment [32,33]. While the therapeutic alliance in guided online interventions is often assumed to be less salient to outcome [9], Flückiger and colleagues [28] have suggested that the overall alliance–outcome association in online therapy is comparable to the association in face-to-face treatment ($r = 0.28$, 95% CI 0.21, 0.34, $p < 0.001$), with higher alliance accompanying better treatment outcomes. A recent review has suggested that the association between alliance and outcome in online interventions may be stronger in terms of agreement on goals and tasks than in terms of the affective bond between patients and their therapists, partly because patients could have lower or different expectations of the bond that can be formed online [32]. In a recent Swedish study ($n = 73$), patients and therapists provided high alliance ratings for blended CBT [34]. The working alliance as rated by therapists, but not as rated by patients, was found predictive of changes in depression severity during treatment. Among the possible explanations for this finding, the authors suggest that therapists in blended cognitive behavioral therapy (bCBT) might have provided more accurate evaluations of working alliance than patients, because patients would have based their alliance ratings on both the online (self-help) material and the face-to-face contacts, whereas therapists would have rated the interaction with the patient in face-to-face contacts only.

The present study expands on existing knowledge by examining working alliance in a randomized controlled trial (RCT), with comparison of blended cognitive behavioral therapy (bCBT) to face-to-face CBT in patients with major depressive disorder (MDD) requiring specialist mental health care. Information on the working alliance was gathered from both patients and therapists, in order to gain insight into the dyadic nature of this relationship [30]. Data was collected in an RCT focusing on the cost-effectiveness of bCBT versus face-to-face CBT [24,35]. The blended intervention integrated face-to-face and online CBT into a single treatment protocol [20,24,35], replacing half of the face-to-face sessions by online sessions. This paper addresses three research questions: (1) Is there a difference between bCBT and face-to-face CBT in terms of patient and therapist ratings of working alliance? (2) Is there an association between working alliance and change in depressive symptoms? and (3) If so, does that association differ between bCBT and face-to-face CBT?

2. Materials and Methods

2.1. Study Design

Data were collected between August 2014 and May 2017 within a pilot randomized controlled trial ($n = 102$), that compared bCBT with face-to-face CBT in six outpatient specialized mental healthcare clinics. The total RCT sample consisted of 102 participants aged 19–62. A detailed overview of the design and procedures of the trial can be found elsewhere [35]. The trial was registered at the Netherlands Trial Register (number NTR4650) and was approved by the Medical Ethics Committee of the Vrije Universiteit Medical Center (VUmc) (registration number 2014.191).

2.2. Participants

Patients for the trial were recruited during the intake procedure before the start of their specialized depression treatment. All patients had a primary diagnosis of MDD, based on the Mini-international Neuropsychiatric Interview Plus (MINI-plus, [36,37]), and had adequate proficiency in the Dutch language, a valid e-mail address, and a computer with Internet access. Patients with a high risk for suicide, a psychotic disorder, a bipolar disorder, or substance dependence were excluded from study participation. No exclusion criteria were applied regarding treatment histories, other comorbidity, or parallel pharmacological treatments. The current study included patients for whom patient-rated or therapist-rated alliance at week 10 was available (n = 92; bCBT n = 45, CBT n = 47).

2.3. Procedures

Patients were asked to provide written informed consent in order to participate in the study. Demographic data, treatment preference, and diagnostic profiles were assessed prior to random allocation and start of treatment (baseline). Working alliance was assessed ten weeks after the start of treatment. At this time point, both groups ideally would have received ten face-to-face sessions. The bCBT group was expected to have received nine additional online sessions and eight online therapist feedback messages. Patients completed weekly assessments on their depression severity during their treatment. Assessments at baseline and after ten weeks of treatment consisted of online self-report questionnaires and a diagnostic interview, administered by trained assessors who were blinded to treatment allocation.

2.4. Random Allocation

Random allocation (1:1 ratio) was performed by an independent researcher, based on a computer-generated random number table. Random allocation was stratified per treatment center. Patients began treatment approximately three weeks after random allocation (SD 2.0, range 0 to 14).

2.5. Interventions

Depression treatment in both study arms was based on CBT manuals [38,39], which advise therapists to provide 15 to 20 weekly CBT sessions and to include psycho-education, behavioral activation, cognitive restructuring, and relapse prevention. The face-to-face CBT without the online sessions was provided at the outpatient clinics. Therapists were advised to plan weekly sessions but were allowed to deviate from the treatment manual when necessary. Duration of treatment could vary per patient, but was expected to last approximately 20 weeks.

Blended CBT consisted of ten face-to-face sessions at the clinic and nine online sessions. Face-to-face and online sessions were alternated. Therapists had received training in the use of the bCBT manual. The aim was to schedule one face-to-face, one online session, and one online feedback message per week during a ten-week period, beginning with a face-to-face session. Patients planned the sessions together with their therapist. Each session focused on a specific domain of the CBT protocol, such as psycho-education, activity scheduling, and identification of dysfunctional assumptions. The content of the online sessions corresponded with that of the previous face-to-face session. Sessions were provided in a fixed order, but therapists were allowed to repeat an online session. In order to access the web-based part of treatment, patients and therapists logged into a personal account on a secure website (www.minddistrict.com). The online sessions consisted of text, short videos, images, patient vignettes, and homework exercises. Patients also had access to a daily mood diary, weekly monitoring of depression severity (QIDS-SR, Quick Inventory of Depressive Symptomatology,

Self-Report version) [40], and a messaging function to contact their therapists. Therapists provided a written therapeutic feedback message to each completed online session. Feedback was asynchronous and was provided within three working days after patients had completed the online session. After reading their therapist's feedback, patients gained access to the next online session. More detailed information on the form and content of bCBT can be found elsewhere [20,35].

2.6. Therapists

A total of 33 therapists participated in the trial, 5 of whom only provided face-to-face CBT, 12 only provided bCBT only, and the remaining 16 therapists treated patients in both treatment arms. On average, therapists treated three patients (SD 2.5, range 1 to 10). All therapists had at least a master's degree in psychology, were specialized in cognitive behavioral treatment, and had a minimum of two years of relevant work experience.

2.7. Measures

In assessing therapeutic alliance, this study focused on Bordin's definition of working alliance [41], which refers to the *bond* between patient and therapist as well as agreement about the *goals* and *tasks* in treatment. Patients and therapists were asked separately to assess their working alliance with the abbreviated Dutch version of the Working Alliance Inventory Short-form Revised (WAI-SR) questionnaire [42–44]. Both questionnaire versions were scored on a five-point Likert scale, ranging from "never" to "always". Items are grouped to measure the three components of working alliance: agreement on Goals, agreement on Tasks, and the quality of the Bond between therapist and patient [41]; a composite (average) score is also calculated as a global assessment of working alliance. Examples of items are "We are working towards mutually agreed upon goals" for the Goal component; "I believe the way we are working with my problem is correct" for the Task component; and "We respect each other" for the Bond component. The client version (WAI-SR-C) consists of 12 items [45], the therapist version (WAI-SR-T) of 10 items. For descriptive purposes, patient and therapist ratings were transformed to a 0 to 5 range for each component. In the current study, both versions of the WAI displayed good internal consistency. Cronbach's alpha for the patient version was 0.91 (95% CI 0.89; 0.94) for the composite score (all items), 0.86 (95% CI 0.82; 0.91) for the Goal component, 0.90 (95% CI 0.86; 0.93) for the Task component, and 0.82 (95% CI 0.77; 0.87) for the Bond component. For the therapist version, Cronbach's alpha was 0.88 (95% CI 0.84; 0.91) for the composite score, 0.81 (95% CI 0.74; 0.87) for the Goal component, 0.81 (95% CI 0.74; 0.87) for the Task component, and 0.79 (95% CI 0.71; 0.85) for the Bond component.

Change in self-reported depression severity was assessed with the Dutch translation of the 16-item short version of the Inventory of Depressive Symptomatology (QIDS-SR) [40]. Patients were requested to complete the QIDS on a weekly basis during treatment. The questionnaire covers all nine components of the DSM-IV-TR (Diagnostic and Statistical Manual of Mental Disorders, fourth edition, text-revision) depression diagnosis. Total scores range between 1 and 27. In the current study, the Cronbach's alpha at baseline was 0.78 (95% CI 0.71; 0.84).

Before random allocation, demographic information, including age, gender, employment status, and income, was collected with an online self-report questionnaire at baseline. One further item was added to inquire whether patients would prefer receiving bCBT or face-to-face CBT. Diagnosis of depression and psychiatric comorbidity were obtained using the Mini-international Neuropsychiatric Interview Plus (MINI-plus, [36,37]). Information on face-to-face treatment uptake (number of sessions completed) was retrieved from patient records. Information on the number of feedback messages received and online sessions completed by patients was obtained from logfiles from the online treatment environment.

2.8. Statistical Analyses

The current study was based on a data subset from a larger trial (n = 102) [24,35], and was therefore not powered a priori. The study sample (N = 92) was large enough to detect a correlation of r ~ 0.3 and a group difference of d ~ 0.6 at a power of 80% and a significance level of p = 0.05.

Multivariable logistic regression analysis including age, gender, partner status, baseline depression severity, comorbidity, treatment group, a priori treatment preference, and total number of face-to-face sessions received was performed to examine possible differences between patients that did and did not provide working alliance ratings.

Between-group differences in patient and therapist ratings of the separate work alliance components were examined using Welch Two-Sample t-test ($p < 0.05$), with patient and therapist ratings as the dependent variable and treatment group as the independent variable.

The degree of consensus between patients and therapists was examined by calculating correlations between patient and therapist ratings. Shapiro–Wilk tests, at alpha = 0.05 [46], revealed non-normal distributions for all separate components, except for the patient ratings on the Task component. We therefore assessed Spearman's rho (for all component pairs. Correlations were estimated using the psych package (version 1.8.4) [47] in R software (Macintosh; Intel Mac OS X v3.5.1) [48]. The relationship between change in depression severity over time, treatment group, and patient- and therapist-rated working alliance was assessed in separate linear mixed-effect models (LMM) with restricted maximum likelihood (REML). The LMM approach was chosen in order to account for missing QIDS data and the correlation between follow-up time points. Because the Goal, Task, and Bond components were moderately to highly intercorrelated (range Task~Bond = 0.41 to Task~Goal = 0.70), only the composite scores were used to examine the association between general working alliance and outcome. The models thus employed QIDS depression severity scores as the independent variable and time (in weeks), treatment group, and the WAI composite scores as dependent variables. Composite scores were centered. The models also included a random effect for individuals over time, which allowed for estimation of individual intercepts and slopes [49,50]. The Holm–Bonferroni correction [51] was applied to account for multiple testing. In the manuscript, noncorrected nonsignificant p-values are reported for descriptive purposes. The mixed models were estimated using the lmer function from the lme4 package (version 1.1–17) [52] in R software (Macintosh; Intel Mac OS X, v3.5.1) [48].

3. Results

3.1. Patients

From the full trial sample of 102 patients (bCBT n = 53, CBT n = 49), data on working alliance was available for 92 patients (bCBT n = 45, CBT n = 47). Both the patient and therapist ratings had been obtained for 71 of them (bCBT n = 38, CBT n = 33), whereas solely therapist ratings were obtained for 19 patients (bCBT n = 8, CBT n = 11) and patient ratings for 2 patients (bCBT n = 1, CBT n = 1). Information on baseline demographic and clinical characteristics of patients included in this study (N = 92) is presented in Table 1.

Table 1. Sample characteristics at baseline.

	bCBT $n = 47$	CBT $n = 45$	Total $n = 92$
Demographic			
Gender, female (n, %)	30 (63.8)	25 (55.6)	43 (59.8)
Age (mean, SD)	39.5 (11.4)	37.7 (10.5)	38.6 (11.0)
In a relationship (n, %)	26 (55.3)	27 (60.0)	53 (57.6)
Education (n, %)			
Low	6 (12.8)	1 (2.2)	7 (7.6)
Middle	24 (51.1)	31 (68.9)	55 (59.8)
High	17 (36.2)	13 (28.9)	30 (32.6)
Employed (n, %)	27 (57.5)	26 (57.8)	53 (57.6)
Nationality, Dutch (n, %)	42 (89.4)	44 (97.8)	68 (93.5)
Clinical			
Treatment preference, bCBT (n, %)	30 (63.8)	30 (66.7)	60 (65.2)
Co-morbid disorder(s) (n, %)	31 (66.0)	30 (66.7)	61 (66.3)
QIDS-SR (mean, SD)	16.6 (4.9)	15.9 (4.1)	16.3 (4.6)
Antidepressant medication (n, %)	32 (68.0)	27 (60.0)	59 (64.1)

Notes: bCBT: blended cognitive behavioral therapy; CBT: cognitive behavioral treatment (face-to-face only); QIDS-SR: Quick Inventory of Depressive Symptomatology, Self-Report version; SD: Standard deviation.

3.2. Study Dropout

Gender, age, relationship status, employment, treatment preference, comorbidity, depression severity, and treatment group were not significantly related to missing working alliance ratings ($p > 0.5$). Patients who received fewer face-to-face sessions during the first ten weeks of treatment had higher odds of not providing information on working alliance ($\beta = -0.849$, OR = 0.43, 95% CI: 0.23; 0.64, $p < 0.001$). In addition, there was a high overlap between study dropout and treatment dropout; six out of nine patients who did not provide data also did not receive any face-to-face sessions.

3.3. Treatment Received

Table 2 provides an overview of treatment received before and after the alliance ratings (ten weeks after start of treatment). Before rating therapeutic alliance, patients in the bCBT group had received an average of 7.1 (SD 2.1) face-to-face sessions and 7.9 (SD 2.4) online sessions; those in the face-to-face CBT group had received a mean of 6.6 (SD 2.2) sessions by week 10. Average per-patient therapist time, including time spent on online feedback, during the first ten weeks of treatment was 636 min (SD 187) in bCBT and 395 min (SD 132) in face-to-face CBT. This difference was statistically significant—95% CI −308.7; −173.5, t (90) = −7.08, Holm-corrected $p < 0.001$. Over the full study period, therapist time between the two groups did not significantly differ (bCBT 944 min SD 274 versus CBT 844 min SD 348, $p = 0.130$). Overall, the face-to-face CBT group received more sessions at the clinic than the bCBT group—14.1 sessions (SD 5.8) versus 11.1 sessions (SD 3.5); mean difference 3.0, 95% CI 1.0; 5.0, t (71.23) = 2.99, $p = 0.004$, Holm-corrected $p = 0.008$).

Table 2. Treatment received in the two study groups.

	bCBT n = 47	CBT n = 45	Total n = 92
Treatment received before assessment of working alliance: mean (SD)			
Face-to-face sessions	7.1 (2.1)	6.6 (2.2)	6.7 (2.2)
Online sessions	7.9 (2.4)	-	-
Online feedback messages	6.9 (2.5)	-	-
Therapist time in minutes	636 (187)	395 (132)	518 (203)
Treatment received after assessment of working alliance: mean (SD)			
Face-to-face sessions	4.0 (2.7)	7.5 (4.8)	5.7 (4.3)
Online sessions	2.7 (2.8)	-	-
Online feedback messages	2.4 (2.6)	-	-
Therapist time in minutes	308 (208)	449 (289)	377 (258)
Treatment received during the full study period: mean (SD)			
Face-to-face sessions	11.1 (3.5)	14.1 (5.8)	12.5 (5.0)
Online sessions	10.3 (2.9)	-	-
Online feedback messages	9.3 (3.5)	-	-
Therapist time in minutes	944 (274)	844 (348)	895 (315)

Notes: bCBT: blended cognitive behavioral therapy; CBT: cognitive behavioral treatment (face-to-face only).

Comparing the total amount of treatment received in both groups with the planned amount of sessions based on the bCBT and CBT treatment protocols, we found that the bCBT group received on average 111% of the planned sessions (averaging one additional face-to-face session and one additional online session) and the CBT group received 70% to 94% (14 out of 15 to 20 planned sessions).

3.4. Working Alliance

After applying a Holm–Bonferroni correction [51] to account for multiple testing, we found no statistically significant differences between treatment groups on either the patient-rated or the therapist-rated composite scores, and also not on the separate Task, Goal, and Bond components of working alliance. Results are shown in Table 3.

Table 3. Patient- and therapist-rated working alliance in the two treatment groups.

	Patients				Therapists			
Outcome [1]	bCBT $n = 39$	CBT $n = 34$	Total $n = 73$	Mean difference (95% CI) bCBT vs. CBT	bCBT $n = 46$	CBT $n = 44$	Total $n = 90$	Mean difference (95% CI) bCBT vs. CBT
Goal	16.3 (3.1)	16.1 (3.2)	16.2 (3.1)	0.25 (−1.22; 1.71)	12.4 (1.9)	11.7 (1.8)	12.1 (1.9)	0.73 (0.04; 1.50) [a]
Scaled	4.1 (0.8)	4.0 (0.8)	4.1 (0.8)		4.1 (0.6)	3.9 (0.6)	4.0 (0.6)	
Task	12.4 (4.1)	11.9 (4.2)	12.2 (4.1)	0.47 (−1.45; 2.40)	12.1 (2.0)	11.2 (1.6)	11.7 (1.9)	0.93 (0.17; 1.68) [b]
Scaled	3.1 (1.0)	3.0 (1.1)	3.0 (1.0)		4.0 (0.7)	3.7 (0.5)	3.9 (0.6)	
Bond	15.6 (3.3)	14.7 (3.6)	15.2 (3.4)	0.97 (−0.64; 2.57)	17.9 (1.9)	17.6 (2.1)	17.7 (2.0)	0.28 (−0.52; 1.17)
Scaled	3.9 (0.8)	3.7 (0.9)	3.8 (0.9)		4.6 (0.5)	4.4 (0.5)	4.4 (0.5)	
Composite	3.7 (0.7)	3.6 (0.8)	3.6 (0.8)	0.14 (−0.22; 0.50)	4.2 (0.5)	4.0 (0.4)	4.1 (0.5)	0.20 (0.00; 0.40) [c]

Notes: [1] Data are presented as mean (standard deviation). bCBT: blended cognitive behavioral therapy; CBT: cognitive behavioral treatment (face-to-face only). [a] uncorrected: $p = 0.063$, Holm-corrected: $p = 0.144$; [b] uncorrected: $p = 0.016$, Holm-corrected: $p = 0.063$; [c] uncorrected: $p = 0.048$, Holm-corrected: $p = 0.424$.

Linear regression analyses showed no significant differences between treatment groups in the associations between patient and therapist evaluations of Task and Goal. In terms of the Bond and the composite scores, positive therapist evaluations appeared to have stronger associations with more positive patient evaluations in the bCBT group, but these were not significant after correction for multiple testing (Bond: 95% CI 0.16; 1.72, $p = 0.019$, Holm-corrected $p = 0.077$; composite: 95% CI −0.0; 1.49; $p = 0.053$, Holm-corrected: $p = 0.160$).

Controlling for therapist time invested in treatment in explorative linear regression analyses led to similar outcomes as described above in the uncontrolled analyses, showing nonsignificant between-group differences in patient-rated alliance, therapist-rated alliance, and associations between patient and therapist evaluations ($p > 0.05$).

In the full sample, patient and therapist composite scores were not significantly related, nor were ratings with regard to the Goal and Bond components. On the Task component, a significant moderate correlation of $\varrho = 0.41$ was found (95% CI: 0.20; 0.59, $p < 0.001$, Holm-corrected $p = 0.001$). In order to gain further insight into the level of agreement between patients and therapists, a difference score was calculated by subtracting the (recoded) therapist composite score from the patient composite score (range 0 to 5). Results showed that 43 out of 71 patients (61%) gave lower ratings than their therapists (mean −1.1, range −2.2 to −0.3); 14 patients (20%) gave similar ratings (mean −0.1, range −0.2 to 0.2), and 11 patients (16%) gave more positive evaluations (mean 0.7, range 0.3 to 4.0).

Explorative linear regression models assessing the relationship between therapist time and the therapist and patient ratings revealed only a significant positive association between therapist time and therapists' ratings of the Task component. This relationship remained significant after controlling for treatment condition (t (85) = 2.84, $p = 0.006$, Holm-corrected $p = 0.023$).

3.5. Working Alliance and Depression Severity

On average, patients completed 22.7 (SD 8.6, range 1 to 42) QIDS measurements. In the week before the assessment of working alliance at ten weeks, the mean QIDS depression severity score was 13.3 (SD 6.2, range 1 to 27), indicating moderately severe depression. Visual inspection of change in depression severity over time suggested a curvilinear pattern. Therefore, linear and quadratic trends were tested in a polynomial model. Adding the polynomial terms to the model led to a better model fit ($p < 0.001$). For patient-rated working alliance (composite score), there was a significant three-way interaction between both the linear and quadratic trends, treatment group and alliance—linear: $b = 0.61$ (95% CI 0.34; 0.88), t (169.50) = 4.25, Holm-corrected $p < 0.001$, quadratic: $b = -0.03$ (95% CI −0.04; −0.02), t (1028) = −5.34, Holm-corrected $p < 0.001$. In Figure 1, the association is visualized by rounding centered alliance scores to low (−1, $n = 21$, range 2.0 to 3.0), medium (0, $n = 32$, range 3.1 to 3.9), and high alliance (1, $n = 21$, range 4.0 to 5.0). Combined with weekly QIDS data, there were 320, 543, and 255 data points available in the respective categories. Density of data points is displayed along the x-axes of the three graphs. The direction of the regression lines after 20 weeks should be interpreted cautiously, because fewer data points were available after that time point.

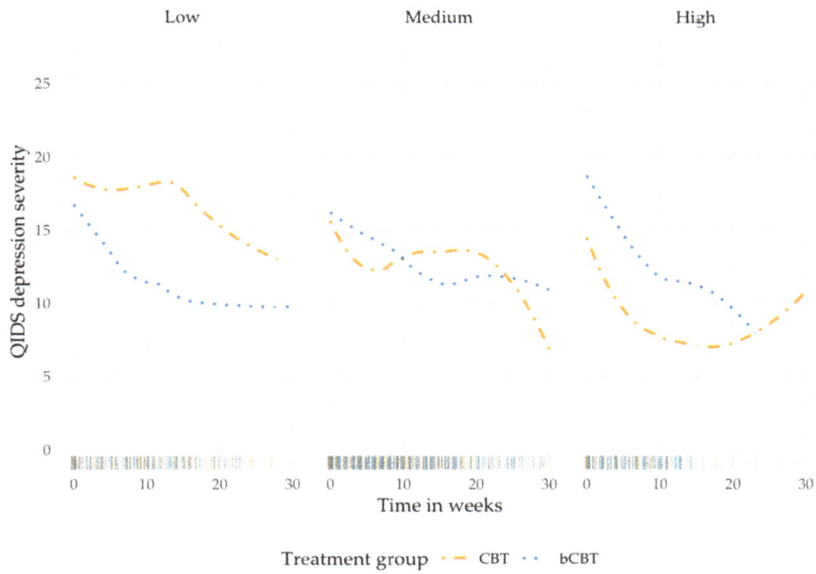

Figure 1. Observed change in depression over time for both treatment groups, clustered in low, medium, and high patient-rated working alliance (measured at week 10). bCBT: blended Cognitive Behavioral Therapy; CBT: Cognitive Behavioral Therapy (face-to-face only); QIDS: Quick Inventory of Depressive Symptomatology.

The graphs in Figure 1 suggest that depression severity in the face-to-face CBT group was associated with patient evaluations of working alliance. In the bCBT group, a similar pattern of decreasing depression severity appeared to occur in all three alliance categories. Post hoc subgroup analyses supported this theory. In bCBT, no alliance–outcome association was found. In the face-to-face CBT group, patients who provided higher ratings had significantly lower QIDS scores—$b = -7.78$ (95% CI −13.10; −1.95), $t\,(27.21) = -2.68$, uncorrected $p = 0.012$—than patients giving lower ratings. Control for therapist time invested in treatment did not alter the findings. Table 4 shows the results of the linear mixed model assessing patient-rated working alliance.

Table 4. Results of the linear mixed model with patient-rated working alliance.

	Dependent Variable				
Predictors	**Estimates**	**SE**	**95% CI**	**Statistic**	***p*-value**
(Intercept)	14.96	0.88	13.25; 16.68	17.08	<0.001
Time × group × working alliance	0.61	0.14	0.33; 0.89	4.25	<0.001
Quadratic time × group × working alliance	−0.03	0.00	−0.04; −0.02	−5.34	<0.001

Notes: SE: Standard error. Random effects: residual (σ^2) = 6.63; intercept (τ_{00}) = 20.70; slope (τ_{11}) = 0.08; intercept–slope covariance (ϱ_{01}) = −0.17; intraclass correlation coefficient (ICC) = 0.76; N = 70; Observations 1118; Marginal R^2/Conditional R^2 = 0.191/0.804; log likelihood = −2861.15.

Therapist-rated alliance was not significantly associated with outcome ($p > 0.05$). LMM revealed similar significant interactions between treatment group and the linear and quadratic trends, suggesting a steeper decrease in depression severity during the first ten weeks of treatment in the bCBT group versus a more linear pattern of decrease of severity in the face-to-face CBT group. Rounding centered alliance scores for descriptive purposes showed that therapists provided lower overall alliance ratings in 2 cases (range 2.9 to 3.0), medium ratings in 58 cases (range 3.1 to 3.9), and high ratings in 30 cases (range 4.0 to 5.0). Explorative analysis revealed no association between the level of agreement (convergence) between patients' and therapists' working alliance ratings and outcome ($p > 0.05$).

4. Discussion

This study examined working alliance between patients and their therapists in blended cognitive behavioral therapy (bCBT) for depression, as provided in specialized mental healthcare settings, and compared it with the working alliance in face-to-face CBT.

4.1. Working Alliance between Patients and Therapists

No differences were found between treatment groups in the way patients and therapists evaluated the working alliance, nor in the associations between patient and therapist ratings of working alliance within either group. This suggests that providing part of treatment online, rather than face-to-face, did not have a negative impact on working alliance between patients and therapists. This is an important finding, because prior research found that therapists voiced this as one of their concerns when considering blended treatment [18]. In general, patients and therapists in both treatment groups were satisfied with the working alliance. Because the current study was one of the first to examine working alliance in bCBT compared with face-to-face CBT, these results cannot be related to outcomes from other studies yet. The high alliance ratings are similar to those reported in other studies that examined patient- and therapist-rated alliance, for example, the trial by Preschl and colleagues ($N = 53$) which compared online CBT with face-to-face CBT for depression [33], and the uncontrolled study by Vernmark and colleagues ($N = 73$) in blended CBT for depression [34].

While both patients and therapists provided positive ratings on average in the current study, no significant association was found between patient and therapist evaluations on general alliance (composite score), and on the Goal and Bond components. On the Task component a moderate positive association was found in the full study sample ($\varrho = 0.41$, 95% CI: 0.20; 0.59), suggesting that higher patient ratings on the Task domain concurred with higher therapist ratings. Further exploration of general working alliance showed that over half of the patients (43 out of 71, 61%) provided less positive evaluations than their therapist, with an average of minus 1 point on a five-point scale. While this is a notable finding, the level of agreement between patients and therapists was not associated with change in depression severity or vice versa. This suggests the degree of convergence after ten weeks of treatment did not impact the treatment effect in the current study.

4.2. Association between Working Alliance and Depressive Symptoms

For patient-rated alliance, an alliance–outcome association was found in the face-to-face group, but not in the bCBT group. In face-to-face CBT, higher depression severity was accompanied by lower alliance ratings, and vice versa. The results for bCBT concurred with the findings of the above-cited study by Vernmark and colleagues [34], which likewise found no alliance–outcome association for patient-rated working alliance in bCBT. That study, however, did not include a comparison group in the analyses. The cause of the disparity in the alliance–outcome association between our study groups cannot be determined here, and more research is needed. Because patients in both groups received CBT, the difference in the alliance–outcome association is more likely to be related to treatment *form* rather than to *content* or therapeutic techniques. One possible explanation is that in bCBT, more emphasis was placed on self-efficacy and autonomy by letting patients work through part of the treatment protocol on their own via the online platform. Hence, patients in bCBT were possibly less dependent on their therapist to achieve a change in depression severity than patients in the face-to-face CBT group.

In this study, no association between therapist-rated alliance and outcome was found in both groups. A possible explanation is that therapists were predominantly positive about the working alliance with their patients, thus restricting variance in this variable and limiting the feasibility of detecting associations between change in depression severity and working alliance. Comparison to other work is complicated, as therapist ratings are often not included in studies. The meta-analytic synthesis by Flückiger and colleagues [28], for example, identified 295 study samples that examined alliance in adult psychotherapy for various mental health problems, but only 40 (14%) of these included therapist ratings. Overall, the synthesis found similar alliance–outcome associations for the alliance ratings of both patients and therapists, suggesting that our current findings are not consistent with general findings on this issue. The same holds for the findings in the Vernmark study, where a significant association was found for therapist ratings and outcome in bCBT, but not for patient ratings, with each point increase in therapist ratings being associated with a 0.5 point reduction per week on the PHQ-9 (Patient Health Questionnaire-9) (95% CI −0.74; −0.26).

4.3. Change in Depressive Symptoms

Over the full study period (30 weeks), both of our treatment groups showed a similar overall improvement in depressive symptoms. Compared with patients in standard face-to-face CBT, those in bCBT reported a steeper decrease in depression severity in the first fifteen weeks of treatment, after which depression scores stabilized. In the face-to-face group, a more linear pattern was observed. This difference is an indication that the higher treatment intensity in bCBT might lead to additional health benefits. Our planning of bCBT treatment intensity was based on the 2013 meta-regression analysis by Cuijpers and colleagues [53], which focused on the amount of psychotherapy required to treat depression. The study suggested that, rather than treatment duration and dosage, the intensity in which sessions are offered per week positively impacts the effect of treatment. While the original goal of providing 18 bCBT sessions in ten weeks [35] was not met in the current study, patients did receive an average of 78% of treatment during that time frame, while those in the less intensive face-to-face CBT group received 37% of the treatment protocol during this period. However, such results should be interpreted with caution, as the current study was not designed to specifically examine the relationship between treatment intensity and treatment effects. Future studies should explore this further, along with the possible role a blended approach could play in achieving higher effectiveness through higher intensity.

4.4. Strengths and Limitations

The current study was one of the first to examine working alliance in a blended cognitive behavioral treatment format in routine practice, and to compare it with alliance in standard face-to-face CBT. By assessing depression severity at a weekly basis, the study also sheds light on the changing severity of depression over the course of treatment, revealing patterns of change rather than absolute differences measured before and after therapy. Moreover, the study included both patient and therapist evaluations of working alliance, providing insights into the degree of convergence between the actors and its possible effects on treatment outcome.

There are also some limitations to be considered while interpreting the results. First, working alliance was treated as a stable factor and was therefore measured only once. That time point was chosen in relation to the expected ten-week duration of the bCBT protocol. Future studies could consider performing an additional measurement at an early stage of treatment, or integrating a weekly assessment of working alliance into the treatment. That would help clarify changes and dynamics in therapeutic alliance over time. Repeated measures would enable more detailed comparison of patterns of depression severity and alliance ratings.

Second, the study had a relatively small sample size, which limited the power to detect small to moderate effects. These have therefore not been revealed by our study. Larger studies could also examine factors that potentially moderate or mediate associations, such as patient demographics, number of prior episodes, and prior experiences with treatment.

Third, the current study specifically focused on patients in outpatient special mental health care for depression. In order to further establish the potential value of bCBT, it is important to evaluate bCBT in other settings, such as primary care, and in different countries. Results from a large European study are forthcoming, examining the comparative effectiveness of bCBT versus treatment as usual in eight different European countries [16].

Additionally, it would be interesting to differentiate between online and face-to-face working alliance within bCBT. Patients might have different expectations of agreement on goals and tasks in the face-to-face sessions than in the online sessions. In the current study, for example, patients and therapists could modify general tasks and goals during their face-to-face sessions, while the content of the online sessions was fixed. Further, it would be interesting to examine whether patients evaluate the online affective bond differently from the bond with their therapist.

Fourth, 16 out of 33 therapists in our study treated patients in both treatment arms, allowing them to compare their experiences with both types of treatment. This could potentially cause bias. Because of the limited sample size, no subgroup analyses were done to examine a possible effect on the evaluation of working alliance when therapists treat patients in both treatment groups.

Finally, because this was one of the first studies to examine bCBT, therapists were relatively inexperienced with the format. It would be interesting to examine whether working alliance ratings in blended treatment increase with the therapists' level of experience.

5. Conclusions

This study shows that bCBT and face-to-face CBT are associated with similarly high working alliance ratings by both patients and therapists when provided to patients with depression in specialized mental health care. Replacing a proportion of the face-to-face sessions with online sessions and online therapist feedback evidently has no negative effect on working alliance and treatment effect. We did find that a more positive evaluation of working alliance was associated with lower depression severity in face-to-face CBT, whereas no such alliance–outcome association was seen in bCBT. The reason for that difference between treatment groups is still unclear. Replication of these results in larger samples to also enable assessment of possible moderators and mediators is warranted.

Author Contributions: All authors were involved in conceptualization, study design, methodology, and writing the original draft. Data curation, L.K. and J.R.; formal analysis, L.K. and J.R.; funding acquisition, P.v.O. and H.R.; project administration, L.K. and J.W.; supervision, J.R., J.W., P.v.O. and H.R.; visualization, L.K. and J.R.; writing—review & editing, L.K., J.W., P.v.O. and H.R. J.R. died in July 2019, before submission of the manuscript. All authors have read and agreed to the published version of the manuscript.

Funding: This study was funded by The Netherlands Organisation for Health Research and Development (ZonMw); project number 837001007, with initial seed funding by the Netherlands Foundation of Health Insurers (Innovatiefonds Zorgverzekeraars); project number B-12-059.

Acknowledgments: In loving memory of Jeroen Ruwaard. The authors gratefully acknowledge the contribution of all therapy participants, research assistants, therapists and all others who contributed to the study.

Conflicts of Interest: The authors declare no conflict of interest. The funders had no role in the design of the study; in the collection, analyses, or interpretation of data; in the writing of the manuscript, or in the decision to publish the results.

References

1. Kessler, R.C.; Chiu, W.T.; Demler, O.; Merikangas, K.R.; Walters, E.E. Prevalence, severity, and comorbidity of 12-month DSM-IV disorders in the National Comorbidity Survey Replication. *Arch. Gen. Psychiatry* **2005**, *62*, 617–627. [CrossRef]
2. Kohn, R.; Saxena, S.; Levav, I.; Saraceno, B. The treatment gap in mental health care. *Bull. World Health Organ.* **2004**, *82*, 858–866. [PubMed]
3. Demyttenaere, K.; Bruffaerts, R.; Posada-Villa, J.; Gasquet, I.; Kovess, V.; Lepine, J.P.; Angermeyer, M.C.; Bernert, S.; de Girolamo, G.; Morosini, P.; et al. Prevalence, severity, and unmet need for treatment of mental disorders in the World Health Organization World Mental Health Surveys. *JAMA* **2004**, *291*, 2581–2590. [PubMed]
4. Bremmer, F.; van Es, M. *Een Analyse van de Verwachte Kosten en Baten Van Ehealth: Blended Behandelen en Begeleiden*; GGZ Nederland: Amersfoort, The Netherlands, 2013.
5. Van't Hof, E.; Cuijpers, P.; Stein, D.J. Self-help and Internet-guided interventions in depression and anxiety disorders: A systematic review of meta-analyses. *CNS Spectr.* **2009**, *14*, 34–40. [PubMed]

6. Cuijpers, P.; Donker, T.; van Straten, A.; Li, J.; Andersson, G. Is guided self-help as effective as face-to-face psychotherapy for depression and anxiety disorders? A systematic review and meta-analysis of comparative outcome studies. *Psychol. Med.* **2010**, *40*, 1943–1957. [CrossRef]
7. Mohr, D.C.; Lyon, A.R.; Lattie, E.G.; Reddy, M.; Schueller, S.M. Accelerating digital mental health research from early design and creation to successful implementation and sustainment. *J. Med. Internet Res.* **2017**, *19*, e153. [CrossRef]
8. Schröder, J.; Berger, T.; Westermann, S.; Klein, J.P.; Moritz, S. Internet interventions for depression: New developments. *Dialogues Clin. Neurosci.* **2016**, *18*, 203–212.
9. Andersson, G.; Cuijpers, P.; Carlbring, P.; Riper, H.; Hedman, E. Guided Internet-based vs. face-to-face cognitive behavior therapy for psychiatric and somatic disorders: A systematic review and meta-analysis. *World Psychiatry* **2014**, *13*, 288–295. [CrossRef]
10. Cuijpers, P.; Riper, H. Internet Interventions for depressive disorders: An overview. *Revista de Psicopatología y Psicol. Clínica* **2014**, *19*, 209–216. [CrossRef]
11. Richards, D.; Richardson, T. Computer-based psychological treatments for depression: A systematic review and meta-analysis. *Clin. Psychol. Rev.* **2012**, *32*, 329–342. [CrossRef]
12. Andrews, G.; Basu, A.; Cuijpers, P.; Craske, M.G.; McEvoy, P.; English, C.L.; Newby, J.M. Computer therapy for the anxiety and depression disorders is effective, acceptable and practical health care: An updated meta-analysis. *J. Anxiety Disord.* **2018**, *55*, 70–78. [CrossRef] [PubMed]
13. Carlbring, P.; Andersson, G.; Cuijpers, P.; Riper, H.; Hedman-Lagerlöf, E. Internet-based vs. face-to-face cognitive behavior therapy for psychiatric and somatic disorders: An updated systematic review and meta-analysis. *Cogn. Behav. Ther.* **2018**, *47*, 1–18. [CrossRef] [PubMed]
14. Cuijpers, P.; Donker, T.; Johansson, R.; Mohr, D.C.; van Straten, A.; Andersson, G. Self-guided psychological treatment for depressive symptoms: A meta-analysis. *PLoS ONE* **2011**, *6*, e21274. [CrossRef] [PubMed]
15. Andersson, G.; Rozental, A.; Shafran, R.; Carlbring, P. Long-term effects of internet-supported cognitive behaviour therapy. *Expert Rev. Neurother.* **2017**, *18*, 21–28. [CrossRef] [PubMed]
16. Kleiboer, A.; Smit, J.; Bosmans, J.; Ruwaard, J.; Andersson, G.; Topooco, N.; Berger, T.; Krieger, T.; Botella, C.; Baños, R.; et al. European COMPARative Effectiveness research on blended Depression treatment versus treatment-as-usual (E-COMPARED): Study protocol for a randomized controlled, non-inferiority trial in eight European countries. *Trials* **2016**, *17*, 387. [CrossRef]
17. Høifødt, R.S.; Lillevoll, K.R.; Griffiths, K.M.; Wilsgaard, T.; Eisemann, M.; Waterloo, K.; Kolstrup, N. The clinical effectiveness of web-based cognitive behavioral therapy with face-to-face therapist support for depressed primary care patients: Randomized controlled trial. *J. Med. Internet Res.* **2013**, *15*, e153. [CrossRef]
18. Van der Vaart, R.; Witting, M.; Riper, H.; Kooistra, L.; Bohlmeijer, E.T.; van Gemert-Pijnen, L.J.E.W.C. Blending online therapy into regular face-to-face therapy for depression: Content, ratio and preconditions according to patients and therapists using a Delphi study. *BMC Psychiatry* **2014**, *14*, 355. [CrossRef]
19. Kenter, R.M.F.; van de Ven, P.M.; Cuijpers, P.; Koole, G.; Niamat, S.; Gerrits, R.S.; Willems, M.; van Straten, A. Costs and effects of Internet cognitive behavioral treatment blended with face-to-face treatment: Results from a naturalistic study. *Internet Interv.* **2015**, *2*, 77–83. [CrossRef]
20. Kooistra, L.C.; Ruwaard, J.; Wiersma, J.E.; van Oppen, P.; van der Vaart, R.; van Gemert-Pijnen, J.E.W.C.; Riper, H. Development and initial evaluation of blended cognitive behavioural treatment for major depression in routine specialized mental health care. *Internet Interv.* **2016**, *4*, 61–71. [CrossRef]
21. Erbe, D.; Eichert, H.-C.; Riper, H.; Ebert, D.D. Blending face-to-face and Internet-based interventions for the treatment of mental disorders in adults: Systematic review. *J. Med. Internet Res.* **2017**, *19*, e306. [CrossRef]
22. Thase, M.E.; Wright, J.H.; Eells, T.D.; Barrett, M.S.; Wisniewski, S.R.; Balasubramani, G.K.; McCrone, P.; Brown, G.K. Improving the efficiency of psychotherapy for depression: Computer-assisted versus standard CBT. *Am. J. Psychiatry* **2018**, *175*, 242–250. [CrossRef] [PubMed]
23. Berger, T.; Krieger, T.; Sude, K.; Meyer, B.; Maercker, A. Evaluating an e-mental health program ("deprexis") as adjunctive treatment tool in psychotherapy for depression: Results of a pragmatic randomized controlled trial. *J. Affect. Disord.* **2018**, *227*, 455–462. [CrossRef] [PubMed]
24. Kooistra, L.C.; Wiersma, J.E.; Ruwaard, J.; Neijenhuijs, K.; Lokkerbol, J.; van Oppen, P.; Smit, F.; Riper, H. Costs and effectiveness of blended versus standard cognitive behavioral therapy for depressed outpatients in routine specialized mental health care: Pilot randomized controlled trial. *J. Med. Internet Res.* **2019**, *21*, e14261. [CrossRef] [PubMed]

25. Wampold, B.E. How important are the common factors in psychotherapy? An update. *World Psychiatry* **2015**, *14*, 270–277. [CrossRef] [PubMed]
26. Horvath, A.O.; Del Re, A.C.; Flückiger, C.; Symonds, D. Alliance in individual psychotherapy. *Psychotherapy* **2011**, *48*, 9–16. [CrossRef]
27. Zilcha-Mano, S. Is the alliance really therapeutic? Revisiting this question in light of recent methodological advances. *Am. Psychol.* **2017**, *72*, 311–325. [CrossRef]
28. Flückiger, C.; Del, A.C.; Wampold, B.E.; Horvath, A.O. The alliance in adult psychotherapy: A meta-analytic synthesis. *Psychotherapy* **2018**, *55*, 316–340. [CrossRef]
29. Cameron, S.K.; Rodgers, J.; Dagnan, D. The relationship between the therapeutic alliance and clinical outcomes in cognitive behaviour therapy for adults with depression: A meta-analytic review. *Clin. Psychol. Psychother.* **2018**, *25*, 446–456. [CrossRef]
30. Laws, H.B.; Constantino, M.J.; Sayer, A.G.; Klein, D.N.; Kocsis, J.H.; Manber, R.; Markowitz, J.C.; Rothbaum, B.O.; Steidtmann, D.; Thase, M.E.; et al. Convergence in patient-therapist therapeutic alliance ratings and its relation to outcome in chronic depression treatment. *Psychother. Res.* **2017**, *27*, 410–424. [CrossRef]
31. Lorenzo-Luaces, L.; Driessen, E.; DeRubeis, R.J.; Van, H.L.; Keefe, J.R.; Hendriksen, M.; Dekker, J. Moderation of the alliance-outcome association by prior depressive episodes: Differential ffects in cognitive-behavioral therapy and short-term psychodynamic supportive psychotherapy. *Behav. Ther.* **2017**, *48*, 581–595. [CrossRef]
32. Berger, T. The therapeutic alliance in internet interventions: A narrative review and suggestions for future research. *Psychother. Res.* **2017**, *27*, 511–524. [CrossRef] [PubMed]
33. Preschl, B.; Maercker, A.; Wagner, B. The working alliance in a randomized controlled trial comparing online with face-to-face cognitive-behavioral therapy for depression. *BMC Psychiatry* **2011**, *11*, 189. [CrossRef] [PubMed]
34. Vernmark, K.; Hesser, H.; Topooco, N.; Berger, T.; Riper, H.; Luuk, L.; Backlund, L.; Carlbring, P.; Andersson, G. Working alliance as a predictor of change in depression during blended cognitive behaviour therapy. *Cogn. Behav. Ther.* **2019**, *48*, 285–299. [CrossRef] [PubMed]
35. Kooistra, L.C.; Wiersma, J.E.; Ruwaard, J.; van Oppen, P.; Smit, F.; Lokkerbol, J.; Cuijpers, P.; Riper, H. Blended vs. face-to-face cognitive behavioural treatment for major depression in specialized mental health care: Study protocol of a randomized controlled cost-effectiveness trial. *BMC Psychiatry* **2014**, *14*, 290. [CrossRef] [PubMed]
36. Sheehan, D.V.; Lecrubier, Y.; Sheehan, K.H.; Amorim, P.; Janavs, J.; Weiller, E.; Hergueta, T.; Baker, R.; Dunbar, G.C. The Mini-International Neuropsychiatric Interview (M.I.N.I.): The development and validation of a structured diagnostic psychiatric interview for DSM-IV and ICD-10. *J. Clin. Psychiatry* **1998**, *59* (Suppl. 2), 22–33, quiz 34–57. [PubMed]
37. Van Vliet, I.M.; De Beurs, E. Het Mini Internationaal Neuropsychiatrisch Interview (MINI). Een kort gestructureerd diagnostisch psychiatrisch interview voor DSM-IV en ICD-10-stoornissen. *Tijdschr. Psychiatr.* **2007**, *49*, 393–397.
38. Bockting, C.L.H.; Huibers, M.J.H. Protocollaire Behandeling Van Patienten Met Een Depressieve Stoornis. In *Protocollaire Behandelingen Voor Volwassenen Met Psychische Klachten 1*; Keijsers, G.P.J., van Minnen, A., Hoogduin, C.A.L., Eds.; Uitgeverij Boom: Amsterdam, The Netherlands, 2011; pp. 251–288. ISBN 9789461057723.
39. Beck, A.T.; Rush, A.J.; Shaw, B.F.; Emery, G. *Cognitive Therapy of Depression*; Guilford: New York, NY, USA, 1979; ISBN 0898620007.
40. Rush, A.J.; Trivedi, M.H.; Ibrahim, H.M.; Carmody, T.J.; Arnow, B.; Klein, D.N.; Markowitz, J.C.; Ninan, P.T.; Kornstein, S.; Manber, R.; et al. The 16-Item Quick Inventory of Depressive Symptomatology (QIDS), clinician rating (QIDS-C), and self-report (QIDS-SR): A psychometric evaluation in patients with chronic major depression. *Biol. Psychiatry* **2003**, *54*, 573–583. [CrossRef]
41. Bordin, E.S. The generalizability of the psychoanalytic concept of the working alliance. *Psychother. Theory, Res. Pract.* **1979**, *16*, 252–260. [CrossRef]
42. Horvath, A.O.; Greenberg, L.S. Development and validation of the Working Alliance Inventory. *J. Couns. Psychol.* **1989**, *36*, 223–233. [CrossRef]
43. Hatcher, R.L.; Gillaspy, J.A. Development and validation of a revised short version of the working alliance inventory. *Psychother. Res.* **2006**, *16*, 12–25. [CrossRef]

44. Stinckens, N.; Ulburghs, A.; Claes, L. De werkalliantie als sleutelelement in het therapiegebeuren: Meting met behulp van de WAV-12, de Nederlandstalige versie. *Tijdschr. Klin. Psychol.* **2009**, *39*, 44–60.
45. Munder, T.; Wilmers, F.; Leonhart, R.; Linster, H.W.; Barth, J. Working alliance inventory-short revised (WAI-SR): Psychometric properties in outpatients and inpatients. *Clin. Psychol. Psychother.* **2010**, *17*, 231–239. [CrossRef] [PubMed]
46. Shapiro, S.S.; Wilk, M.B. An analysis of variance test for normality (complete samples). *Biometrika* **1965**, *52*, 591–611. [CrossRef]
47. Revelle, W. *Psych: Procedures for Psychological, Psychometric and Personality Research*; Northwestern University: Evanston, IL, USA, 2018.
48. R Core Team. *R: A Language and Environment for Statistical Computing*; R Core Team: Vienna, Austria, 2017.
49. Hesser, H. Modeling individual differences in randomized experiments using growth models: Recommendations for design, statistical analysis and reporting of results of internet interventions. *Internet Interv.* **2015**, *2*, 110–120. [CrossRef]
50. White, I.R.; Carpenter, J.; Horton, N.J. Including all individuals is not enough: Lessons for intention-to-treat analysis. *Clin. Trials* **2012**, *9*, 396–407. [CrossRef]
51. Holm, S. A simple sequentially rejective multiple test procedure. *Scand. J. Stat.* **1979**, *6*, 65–70.
52. Bates, D.; Maechler, M.; Bolker, B.; Walker, S.; Christensen, R.H.B.; Singmann, H.; Dai, B.; Eigen, C. *Linear Mixed-Effects Models using "Eigen" and S4; R package, version 1-1.21*; 2017.
53. Cuijpers, P.; Huibers, M.; Ebert, D.D.; Koole, S.L.; Andersson, G. How much psychotherapy is needed to treat depression? A metaregression analysis. *J. Affect. Disord.* **2013**, *149*, 1–13. [CrossRef]

Journal of
Clinical Medicine

MDPI

Article

Using the Personalized Advantage Index for Individual Treatment Allocation to Blended Treatment or Treatment as Usual for Depression in Secondary Care

Nadine Friedl [1,*], Tobias Krieger [1], Karine Chevreul [2], Jean Baptiste Hazo [3], Jérôme Holtzmann [4], Mark Hoogendoorn [5], Annet Kleiboer [6], Kim Mathiasen [7,8], Antoine Urech [9], Heleen Riper [10,11,12] and Thomas Berger [1]

1 Department of Clinical Psychology, University of Bern, 3012 Bern, Switzerland
2 URC Eco Ile-de-France (AP-HP), Hotel Dieu, 1, Place du Parvis Notre Dame, 75004 Paris, France
3 Eceve, Unit 1123, Inserm, University of Paris, Health Economics Research Unit, Assistance Publique-Hôpitaux de Paris, 75004 Paris, France
4 University Hospital Grenoble Alpes, Mood Disorders and Emotional Pathologies Unit, Pôle de Psychiatrie, Neurologie et Rééducation Neurologique, 38043 Grenoble, France
5 Department of Computer Science, VU University Amsterdam Faculty of Sciences, De Boelelaan 1081m, 1081 HV Amsterdam, The Netherlands
6 Section Clinical Psychology, Faculty of Behavioural and Movement Sciences, Vrije Universiteit Amsterdam and EMGO+ Institute for Health Care and Research, Van der Boechorststraat 1, 1081 BT Amsterdam, The Netherlands
7 Department of Psychology, Faculty of Health Sciences, University of Southern Denmark, 5230 Odense M, Denmark
8 Center of Telepsychiatry, University of Southern Denmark, 5000 Odense, Denmark
9 INSELSPITAL, University Hospital Bern, University Clinic for Neurology, University Acute-Neurorehabilitation Center. 3010 Bern, Switzerland
10 Department of Psychiatry and the Amsterdam Public Health Research Institute, GGZ inGeest/Amsterdam UMC, Vrije Universiteit, de Boelelaan 1117, 1081 HV Amsterdam, The Netherlands
11 Department of Research and Innovation, GGZ inGeest Specialized Mental Health Care, Oldenaller 1, 1081 HJ Amsterdam, The Netherlands
12 Department of Clinical, Neuro-and Developmental Psychology and the Amsterdam Public Health Research Institute, Vrije Universiteit Amsterdam, van der Boechorststraat 7, 1081 BT Amsterdam, The Netherlands
* Correspondence: nadine.friedl@psy.unibe.ch

Received: 30 December 2019; Accepted: 5 February 2020; Published: 11 February 2020

Abstract: A variety of effective psychotherapies for depression are available, but patients who suffer from depression vary in their treatment response. Combining face-to-face therapies with internet-based elements in the sense of blended treatment is a new approach to treatment for depression. The goal of this study was to answer the following research questions: (1) What are the most important predictors determining optimal treatment allocation to treatment as usual or blended treatment? and (2) Would model-determined treatment allocation using this predictive information and the personalized advantage index (PAI)-approach result in better treatment outcomes? Bayesian model averaging (BMA) was applied to the data of a randomized controlled trial (RCT) comparing the efficacy of treatment as usual and blended treatment in depressive outpatients. Pre-treatment symptomatology and treatment expectancy predicted outcomes irrespective of treatment condition, whereas different prescriptive predictors were found. A PAI of 2.33 PHQ-9 points was found, meaning that patients who would have received the treatment that is optimal for them would have had a post-treatment PHQ-9 score that is two points lower than if they had received the treatment that is suboptimal for them. For 29% of the sample, the PAI was five or greater, which means that a substantial difference between the two treatments was predicted. The use of the PAI approach for clinical practice must be further confirmed in prospective research; the current study supports the identification of specific interventions favorable for specific patients.

Keywords: personalized advantage index; depression; blended treatment; CBT; treatment selection; Bayesian model averaging

---

1. Introduction

Globally, 300 million people of all ages suffer from depression [1]. Depression is one of the most common problems seen in clinical practice, and it is associated with high societal costs, as well as great suffering [2]. Given this burden, the need for improved access to efficacious and cost-effective treatments is essential [3]. In the last decades, research has focused on examining different treatment options for depression. Especially, cognitive behavior therapy (CBT) and interpersonal therapy (IPT) can be seen as first-line treatments [4,5]. Moreover, current studies are aimed at scaling up treatments for depression. One way to do so is through internet-based therapies [5]. Whereas the most dominant format in which treatment is delivered is through face-to-face contact, internet-based therapies have received much attention in recent years [6]. The efficacy and cost-effectiveness of the latter have been supported by a growing number of research [7–9]. Even though only a few studies have directly compared internet-based with face-to-face CBT for depression, results suggest it to have similar overall effects [6].

A newer approach to depression treatment is to combine web-based technologies with face-to-face therapy, called blended treatment. Blended treatment includes any combination of face-to-face therapy and internet-based interventions, e.g., web-based components are used as an adjunctive intervention or are integrated during face-to-face therapy [10]. Although research that investigates the efficacy of blended treatment formats is still scarce, preliminary results suggest their feasibility and their efficacy in reducing symptoms of depression [11–15]. For example, a randomized controlled trial by Berger and colleagues [16] showed the superiority of blended treatment, consisting of an internet-based intervention as an adjunct to face-to-face psychotherapy, in comparison to regular face-to-face psychotherapy in a pragmatic randomized controlled study in patients with a unipolar affective disorder in routine care. Another recent study showed the noninferiority of blended treatment to conventional CBT for patients with depression and found blended treatment to be cost-effective [17]. Moreover, the blended treatment has also been evaluated in an inpatient setting where patients suffering from depression that received an online self-help program in addition to inpatient psychotherapy improved significantly more than patients who received online information about depression in addition to inpatient psychotherapy [18]. Furthermore, a recent systematic review showed that, compared to face-to-face therapy, a blended treatment may help maintaining initially achieved changes within psychotherapy in the long-term [19].

Potential benefits of blending treatments may be a greater reduction in depressive symptoms and increased cost-effectiveness [20], as well as an improvement of patients' adherence to the treatment program [21]. Furthermore, an asset of a blended treatment may be that it combines the advantages of both treatment forms [3,14,22,23]. For example, the face-to-face contact enables clinicians to individualize or tailor the treatment and to react in crisis situations, while providing online modules between sessions could promote patient engagement and enhance the translation of treatment into daily life (e.g., [24]). On the other hand, when online components are not used by the patients in blended treatments, reductions in the number of face-to-face sessions may lead to worse treatment outcomes [25]. Furthermore, therapists may raise concerns of overburdening depressed patients [18]. So far, it is not clear for which patients blended treatment may be a feasible option and for which patients a conventional treatment should be favored.

Patients with depression may differ substantially from each other, and evidence suggests that the diagnostic categories leave room for great diversity [26,27]. This results in differences with regard to patients' illness courses and individual treatment responses [28]. Research suggests that individual patient characteristics may moderate the efficacy of different treatments at an individual level [29]. It is, therefore, important to recognize that no single treatment is likely to be the best for everyone, even though, on a group level, it is efficacious for patients suffering from depression [26,30]. This is why more and more researchers move away from investigating treatment efficacy on a group level and instead focus on custom-tailoring the treatment to the individual patient [30,31]. In this sense, it may be a solution to increase the overall treatment response rates [32].

Precision medicine tries to tailor treatments to the specific needs of the patient [33]. More recently, in clinical psychology and psychotherapy, algorithms are used that predict from which treatment a patient benefits the most [34]. As an example, Becker and colleagues [35] introduce a conceptual framework that helps classifying applications of predictive modeling in mental health research. These authors try to bridge the gap between psychologists and predictive modelers with providing a common language for classifying predictive modeling mental health research. They suggest that e-mental health researchers should focus more on the validity of model predictions instead of solely focusing on identifying predictors. Another example is the personalized advantage index PAI) approach, which identifies patients with a certain disorder (e.g., major depression) who benefit more from one treatment than another [30]. Using the personalized advantage index (PAI), it is possible to identify the treatment that predicts a better treatment outcome for a given patient if there are two comparably effective treatments to choose from [36]. The PAI estimates how much a specific treatment is better for an individual patient than another, and its feasibility and relevance have been shown in several studies on the treatment of depression [36–40]. Baseline patient characteristics can be divided into two types of predictors: a prognostic variable predicts treatment outcome irrespective of treatment condition, whereas a prescriptive variable predicts a differential treatment response to two or more treatment modalities [29,30]. Up to today, different treatments have been compared using the PAI, and its values range from 1.4 when comparing CBT to CBT with integrated exposure and emotion-focused elements [38] up to 8.9 when comparing cognitive therapy to IPT [40]. Higher absolute values of the PAI stand for stronger predicted benefits of one treatment over another. Being able to identify the best treatment for an individual with depression is essential, because it may make health care delivery more efficient [32]. Even though predictive modeling is still very young in the field of e-mental health [41], Bremer and colleagues [42] were able to predict clinical outcomes and costs of patients with depression prior to starting blended psychotherapy in a subsample of the current study using machine learning techniques.

In the current study, treatment as usual (TAU), i.e., regular face-to-face psychotherapy, was compared to blended treatment for patients with major depressive disorder (MDD) in secondary care. The present study set out to answer the following research questions: (1) What are the most important predictors determining optimal treatment allocation to TAU or blended treatment? and (2) Would model-determined treatment allocation using this predictive information and the PAI-approach result in better treatment outcomes? To the best of our knowledge, this is the first study comparing different treatment delivering formats, i.e., traditional face-to-face CBT versus blended CBT, by using the PAI-approach.

2. Materials and Methods

Data used in the present study was drawn from the European project "European COMPARative effectiveness research on blended depression treatment" (E-COMPARED, February 2018) [43]. The E-COMPARED project included a randomized, controlled, noninferiority trial that examined the clinical and cost-effectiveness of blended treatment compared to treatment as usual in routine care in nine European countries. Adult patients diagnosed with MDD were recruited in primary or in specialized mental health care. The current study uses the data of the four countries that recruited patients in specialized mental health care (France, the Netherlands, Switzerland, and Denmark). The following inclusion criteria were met by participants: (1) being 18 years of age or older, (2) meeting Diagnostic and Statistical Manual of Mental Disorders (DSM-IV) diagnostic criteria for MDD as confirmed by a telephone-administered MINI international neuropsychiatric interview (M.I.N.I.) version 5.0 [44], and (3) minimal to severe symptoms of depression based on a score of 5 or above on the patient health questionnaire-9 (PHQ-9) [45]. Exclusion criteria for participating in the study were: (1) high risk for suicide according to the M.I.N.I.; (2) psychiatric comorbidity such as substance dependence, bipolar affective disorder, psychotic illness, or obsessive compulsive disorder; (3) currently receiving another psychological treatment for depression; (4) being unable to comprehend the spoken and written language of the country where the study is conducted; (5) not having access to a computer with fast internet connection; and (6) not having a smartphone that is compatible with the mobile component of the intervention that is offered. Patients were randomized to blended treatment or TAU using an allocation scheme with a computerized random number generator at an allocation ratio of 1:1 and between 8 and 14 allocations per block. Details about the study design are described elsewhere [43]. For Switzerland, this study was approved by the cantonal ethics committees Bern and Zurich (registration number: 001/15; date: 18 March 2015); for Denmark, the study was approved by the Ethics Committee of the Region of Southern Denmark (registration number S-20150150; date: 18 November 2015); for France, the study was approved by the "Comité de protection des personnes", Ile de France V (registration number 15033-*n*° 2015-A00565-44; date: 2 June 2015); and, for the Netherlands, the study was approved by the METC VUMC (registration number 2015.078; date: 8 May 2015). Furthermore, all participants provided written informed consent and gave permission to all E-COMPARED partners to use their anonymized data.

2.1. Sample

The current study has a sample size of $n = 251$. The sample consists of 83 participants from the Netherlands (33.9%), 79 participants from France (32.2%), 44 from Switzerland (18.0%), and 39 participants from Denmark (15.9%). The mean age at baseline was 41.0 years (SD = 13.7), and 68.2% of the participants were female. The majority were either single (33.5%) or married (31.8%), and 21.2% of participants were living together and 12.8% were divorced. In the TAU condition, 57.9% of the sample suffered from a recurrent depression, 45.2% from a current melancholic depressive episode, 7.9% from a comorbid dysthymia, and 46.8% from a comorbid anxiety disorder. The number of patients are taking antidepressant medication at the time of the baseline measurement was 53.2%. In the blended treatment condition, 53.8% of the participants suffered from a recurrent depression, 34.5% from a current melancholic depressive episode, 5.9% from a comorbid dysthymia, and 61.3% had a comorbid anxiety disorder. Half of the participants (49.6%) were taking antidepressant medication at baseline.

2.2. Interventions

Individual face-to-face CBT was combined with internet-based CBT elements delivered through a platform for blended treatment. Three different online platforms were used across the participating countries. Switzerland used "Deprexis" [46], whereas Denmark used NoDep [47] and France and the Netherlands used the platform "Moodbuster" [3]. The most important components of the treatment were cognitive restructuring, behavioral activation, psychoeducation, and relapse prevention, which were delivered over 11–20 sessions. In the blended treatment, a smaller number of face-to-face sessions is offered, and some sessions are replaced by online modules. Treatment was provided by CBT therapists who received special training on how to deliver the blended treatment. In Switzerland and the Netherlands, the therapists were either licensed CBT therapists or CBT therapists who were supervised by an experienced licensed CBT therapist. In Denmark, the treatment was delivered by either licensed psychologists or psychologists under supervision of licensed psychologists. In France, the blended treatment was provided by licensed psychotherapists [43].

The TAU treatment was defined as the routine care that patients received in specialized mental health care when they were diagnosed with depression. In practice, this meant that the TAU group received regular fact-to-face CBT.

2.3. Measures

2.3.1. Primary Outcome

The primary outcome measure for this study was the PHQ-9 [45] assessed after 12 weeks. The PHQ-9 consists of nine questions which are based upon the DSM-IV criteria for the diagnosis of depressive disorders. It is used as a diagnostic instrument and as a severity measure for depression. A 5-point difference in PHQ-9 scores is seen as clinically significant [48]. The validity and sensitivity to change of the PHQ-9 were satisfactory in previous studies [49,50]. Cronbach's alpha in the present study was 0.78.

2.3.2. Predictor Variables

We used an exploratory approach and included a total of 28 potential predictors measured at baseline in the analysis. All variables of the baseline assessment that did not exceed a number of acceptable missing values (<50%) were included. We classified the variables into four categories: (1) sociodemographic variables, (2) symptomatology and quality of life, (3) healthcare utilization, and (4) patient expectancy.

The sociodemographic variables included age, marital status, education, gender, and country and were assessed with single item questions. Variables related to symptomatology and treatment history were recurrent depression, therapy preference, dysthymia, melancholic depressive episodes, comorbid anxiety, and current use of antidepressants. Quality of life was measured with the EQ-5D [51]. Healthcare utilization was assessed with the TiC-P [52]. The TiC-P examines healthcare consumption and productivity losses as a consequence of a mental disorder via a self-report questionnaire. The questions include contacts within the healthcare sector and the use of medication. All the questions aim at the period of the last four months before the start of the treatment (see Table 1 for the items of the TiC-P that have been included). Patient expectancy was measured by the credibility and expectancy questionnaire (CEQ; [53]).

Table 1. TiC-P items included in the analysis.

"How many times did you consult a general practitioner?" "How many times did you consult a psychologist?" "How many times did you consult a psychotherapist?", "How many times did you consult a psychiatrist?", and "How many times did you consult a professional from an ambulatory mental health institution?" "How many times did you consult a professional from a clinic for alcohol or drugs?" and "How many times did you consult self-help groups?"	"How many days did you spend in a day-time treatment program in a regular hospital?" "How many days did you spend in a day-time treatment program in a psychiatric hospital?" and "How many days did you use outpatient psychotherapeutic services in addition to your psychotherapy?"	"How many admissions to a regular hospital did you have?" and "How many admissions to a psychiatric hospital did you have?" "How many admissions to a rehabilitation clinic did you have?" "Do you have a paid job?" "Did health problems oblige you to call in sick from work at any time?"

2.4. Data Analytical Strategy

Regarding the predictor variables, a bottom-up approach was followed, which means that even though some variables might have a particular relevance to one treatment or the other, the predictors are treated equally in the data analysis.

2.4.1. Missing Data

In line with previous research using the PAI approach, we included those participants for which PHQ-9 scores after 12 weeks were available [36,38,40]. This left us with n = 245, representing 97.6% of the total sample. Distributed over the two conditions, there were 126 patients in the TAU condition and

119 patients in the blended treatment condition. With regard to the baseline measures, missing values were found in the dimensions credibility and expectancy of the CEQ (3.7% respectively 4.1%), the EQ-5D (1.6%), antidepressants (1.2%), prior psychotherapy (40.4%), comorbid melancholic episodes (14.3%), comorbid dysthymia (5.3%), comorbid anxiety (2.4%), and some items of the TiC-P (2.0–40.8%). We imputed these missings in the baseline measures with the R *missForest* [54]. Here, missing values are predicted on the basis of a random forest approach, trained on observed values of the available data. An advantage of *missForest* is that it imputes categorical and continuous variables simultaneously [55]. It has been shown to be highly accurate and to outperform other imputation methods due to its small imputation error [56]. The imputed data set is the basis for all analyses that follow.

2.4.2. Bayesian Model Averaging (BMA)

There are different data analysis approaches that can be used to identify baseline variables that predict outcome in one treatment versus another. Data analysis approaches that rely on one model only can only include a limited number of baseline measures that could be predictors. In that case, the most common rule that is used states that at least 10 observations per predictor are necessary to not exceed a level of bias which is acceptable [57,58]. If we had followed this approach, we could have only included a small number of predictors. Furthermore, the problem with relying upon a single selected model is that it may result in overconfidence in the conclusions drawn regarding quantified associations. The problem is that there may be alternative models that have different subsets of predictors that fit the data just as well as the one selected model [59,60]. Overfitted models cause uncertainty regarding the actual value of findings, because they may not replicate in future samples [61]. Bayesian model averaging (BMA) is a method that can account for model uncertainty while providing a better predictive ability. The BMA method has two advantages. First, it results in predictions that are less risky and. second, BMA provides simpler model choice criteria, because it uses the Bayesian inference for model prediction and selection [62]. With BMA, a posterior probability is estimated on the basis that each considered model is the correct one. This included the aforementioned model uncertainty in the estimates for the parameter and inferences. That means that BMA averages over all possible predictor sets and delivers model choice criteria that help to identify the most probable model. With using BMA, sharper predictions can be derived from the data, especially in cases with many possible predictors but a limited sample size. Several studies have supported BMA's predictive performance [60,63–66].

The data frame was divided into two subsets: the TAU condition and the blended treatment condition. Using the R package *BAS*, for each condition, a separate linear regression model was computed [67]. Then, Bayesian adaptive sampling (BAS) without replacement for variable selection in linear models using the function *bas.lm* with treatment outcome was applied (PHQ-9 score after 12 weeks) as the dependent variable. The relative importance of each variable was evaluated using the posterior probabilities that were calculated for each potential predictor. The marginal posterior inclusion probabilities functioned as the criteria for determining the importance of the potential predictors. Values above 0.5 point out that the predictor has been incorporated in more than half the models; thus, in the present study, in over 15,000 models. The nominal variables were split into their different categories, which enabled a precise interpretation of the results. The model performance was further evaluated using posterior probabilities. The appropriate *bas.lm* function was chosen based on the following considerations: a Laplace approximation to the Jeffreys-Zellner-Siow (JZS) prior for the integration of alpha = 1 was used as the criterion for the priors, which is called the "ZS-null". The JZS prior uses the Zellner-Siow Cauchy prior on the coefficients and the Jeffreys prior on sigma. The squared scale of the prior, where the default is alpha = 1, can be controlled using the optional parameter "alpha" [38,67]. Marginal inclusion probabilities were calculated with the "MCMC+BAS" method, which runs an initial Markov chain Monte Carlo (MCMC) algorithm and then samples without replacement, as in BAS. Compared to the BAS alone, the "MCMC+BAS" method is the preferred option, because it provides estimates with low bias [68]. The number of models was set to 30,000 assuming that each additional model would add only a small increment to the cumulative probability, i.e., not leading to essential differences in posterior distributions. Due to the limited sample size, the models have been built and tested in the same dataset.

2.4.3. Personalized Advantage Index (PAI)

When predicting the therapy outcome for each patient, applying a leave-one-out approach ("jackknife") to estimate regression models is an essential beginning step in generating the PAI [36,38,69]. In this procedure, overfitting can be avoided by excluding each target patient for whom the PAI prediction is estimated from the model. For each patient, two regression models were built using the treatment-specific predictors identified with BMA. For each patient, a factual prediction (PHQ-9 score at 12 weeks of the treatment the patient has received) and a counterfactual prediction (PHQ-9 score at 12 weeks of the intervention the patient did not receive) were estimated. In the next step, those two predictions were compared, and the prediction that resulted in the best outcome for the patient was defined to be the optimal treatment for that patient. When comparing the observed change scores, the size of the predicted difference of receiving the treatment with the greater predicted benefit is ultimately the PAI [36]. The higher the absolute values of the PAI, the stronger is the predicted benefit of one treatment over another. The interpretation of the PAI can be demonstrated with a recent study that used the PHQ-9 as the primary outcome and found a PAI of 2.5 [70]. This means that if patients had received their "optimal" treatment (out of the two), their PHQ-9 score at 12 weeks would have been 2.5 points lower than if they had obtained their nonoptimal treatment.

3. Results

Henceforth, we firstly report the five best models for each treatment condition, and, secondly, we report the PAI results. The best models are defined based on the highest posterior probability and the lowest Bayesian information criterion (BIC).

3.1. Variables Predicting Outcome in TAU

The five best models predicting depression severity at 12 weeks in the TAU condition are displayed in Table 2. The Bayes factor, number of predictors, R^2, log marginal likelihood, and the posterior probabilities are provided for each model. Model 1 has the largest Bayes factor and the largest posterior probability (0.02) and, thus, seems to fit the data best. As a result, Model 1 was selected as our final predictive model of the PHQ-9 score at 12 weeks in the TAU condition.

Table 2. Five best models for treatment as usual (TAU).

Fit Indices	Model 1	Model 2	Model 3	Model 4	Model 5
Bayes Factor	1	0.934	0.597	0.572	0.510
Number of Variables	6	6	6	5	6
R^2	0.428	0.445	0.441	0.440	0.439
Log Marginal Likelihood	22.729	22.659	22.213	22.170	22.056
Posterior Probabilities	0.021	0.019	0.012	0.012	0.011

While the selected model includes six variables in total, the strongest predictors of the PHQ-9 score at 12 weeks in the TAU condition included the pretreatment PHQ-9 score (Prob = 100%), CEQ expectancy (Prob = 97%), "How many days did you use outpatient psychotherapeutic services in addition to your psychotherapy?" (Prob = 95%), "How many times did you consult a psychiatrist?" (Prob = 64%), Denmark (Prob = 58%), and "How many days did you attend a day-time treatment program in a psychiatric hospital?" (Prob = 51%). A higher pretreatment score, more consultations with a psychiatrist, and more days in a day-time treatment program in a psychiatric hospital prior to treatment predicted a higher PHQ-9 score at 12 weeks. Higher expectancy scores, receiving TAU in Denmark, and more days using outpatient psychotherapeutic services in addition to the psychotherapy prior to treatment predicted lower PHQ-9 scores at 12 weeks. The effects of other variables appeared minimal due to their small posterior probabilities. See Appendix 1 in the Supplemental Online Material for the complete list of variables and their inclusion probabilities.

3.2. Variables Predicting Outcome in the Nlended Treatment

Table 3 gives an overview of the five best models to predict treatment outcome in the blended treatment condition. Based on the posterior probabilities and the Bayes factor, Model 1 was rated the best model. Thus, Model 1 was selected as the final predictive model for the blended treatment condition.

Table 3. Five best models for the blended treatment condition.

Fit Indices	Model 1	Model 2	Model 3	Model 4	Model 5
Bayes Factor	1	0.887	0.577	0.525	0.516
Number of Variables	6	5	4	6	6
R^2	0.398	0.416	0.392	0.429	0.446
Log Marginal Likelihood	19.852	19.731	19.301	19.207	19.190
Posterior Probabilities	0.012	0.011	0.007	0.006	0.006

Based on the posterior probabilities, the most important predictors for treatment outcome in the blended treatment were the pretreatment PHQ-9 score (Prob = 99.9%), regular hospital admissions (Prob = 99.9%), EQ-5D quality of life (Prob = 74.6%), CEQ expectancy (Prob = 72.3%), consulting self-help groups (Prob = 70.0%), and being widowed (Prob = 49.7%). CEQ credibility reached a posterior probability of 42.9%. A higher pretreatment PHQ-9 score, being widowed, more hospital admissions, and consulting self-help groups predicted higher PHQ-9 scores at 12 weeks. A higher expectancy for improvement and a higher quality of life predicted lower PHQ-9 scores after 12 weeks. See Appendix 2 in the Supplemental Online Material for the posterior probabilities of all variables measured at baseline.

3.3. Personalized Advantage Index

Using the treatment specific predictors described above, the prediction of a patient's PHQ-9 score after 12 weeks was computed separately for each treatment condition. The true error of the PHQ-9 score predictions at 12 weeks was 4.16, representing the average absolute difference between the predicted and actual, observed scores across all patients. Patients who were categorized as having received their optimal treatment had a mean PHQ-9 score of 9.67 (n = 124) at 12 weeks, whereas patients who were classified as having received their suboptimal treatment had a mean PHQ-9 score of 12.00 (n = 121). Figure 1 shows the frequency of predicted PHQ-9 scores at 12 weeks for every patient in both the optimal and suboptimal treatments.

In the first step, an individual PAI was calculated for each patient. Secondly, the average PAI was calculated as the mean difference in PHQ-9 scores between the optimal and the suboptimal treatments for each patient. The average PAI of the current study was 2.33. The PAI can be read as follows: if patients had received the treatment that is "optimal" for them, their PHQ-9 score at 12 weeks would have been 2.33 points lower than if they had received the treatment that is suboptimal for them. In Figure 2, the frequencies of the individual PAIs are shown. A PAI that is five or greater would mean that a substantial difference was predicted between the two treatments, because 5 points on the PHQ-9 stands for a minimal clinically meaningful difference for individual change [71]. This was the case for 29% of the patients in this sample.

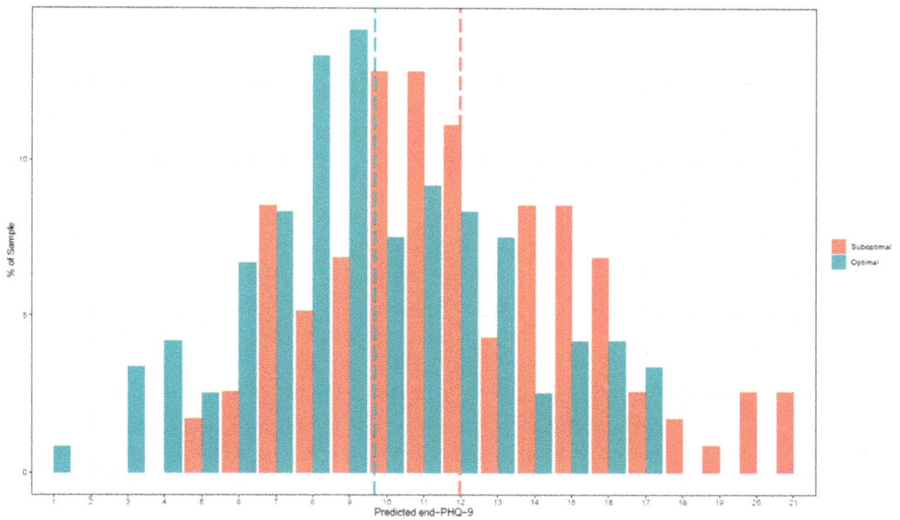

Figure 1. Frequency of predicted PHQ-9 scores at 12 weeks.

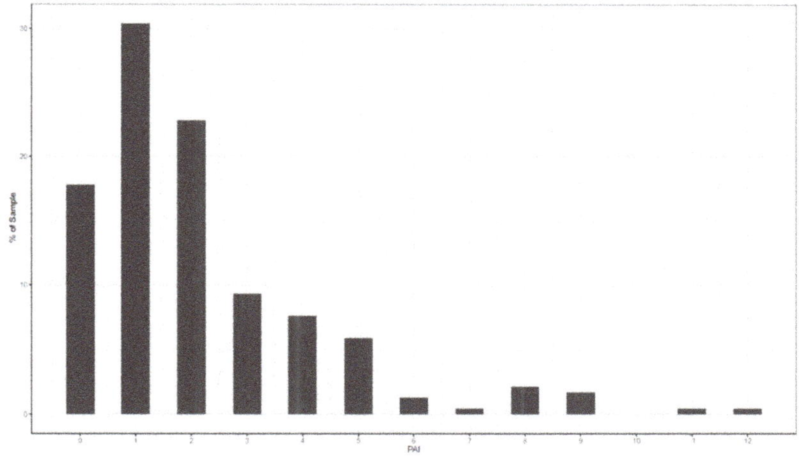

Figure 2. Frequencies of individual personalized advantage indexes (PAIs).

4. Discussion

Regarding the predictors of treatment outcome at 12 weeks in each of the interventions, different relevant predictors were identified for TAU and the blended treatment, respectively. In the TAU condition, a lower pretreatment PHQ-9 score, less consultations with a psychiatrist and less days in a day-time treatment program in a psychiatric hospital, higher expectancy, receiving TAU in Denmark, and more days using outpatient psychotherapeutic services in the four months prior to the study predicted a better treatment outcome, i.e., a lower PHQ-9 score (at 12 weeks). In contrast, in the blended treatment condition, a lower pretreatment PHQ-9 score, not being widowed, less hospital admissions and consulting self-help, a higher expectancy for improvement, and a higher EQ-5D score predicted lower scores at 12 weeks; thus, a better treatment outcome.

To offer an initial interpretation of our findings, the distinction between prescriptive and prognostic predictors is used. Prognostic variables predict treatment outcomes regardless of treatment conditions [30,38]. In contrast, prescriptive variables may support differential indications by predicting whether a patient will benefit more from one treatment in comparison to another. In the present study, the pretreatment depressive symptomatology and treatment expectancy are the only prognostic predictors, i.e., the only variables that predict treatment outcome in both conditions. This is in line with previous research that has found pretreatment symptomatology and expectancy to be important predictors of treatment outcome, in the sense that higher symptomatology before treatment predicts worse end-state symptomatology [30,34,36,38,72,73] and higher expectancy for improvement predicts better treatment outcome [74,75]. Interestingly, for internet-based treatments, higher baseline symptomatology is not necessarily a negative predictor of treatment outcome. More often the opposite is found, i.e., that higher depressive symptomatology pretreatment predicts better treatment outcomes [76–78]. This might be partly explained by the efficacy nature of previous randomized controlled trials (RCTs) in comparison to the routine care and effectiveness nature of the current study.

Regarding the prescriptive predictors, our findings partly corroborate findings from previous studies predicting treatment outcomes for patients with depression. With regard to prescriptive predictors of the blended treatment condition, a lower quality of life and being widowed predicted worse treatment outcomes. In contrast to the present result, the study by Huibers and colleagues [40] found a higher quality of life to be a prognostic predictor, i.e., to predict favorable outcomes irrespective of treatment conditions.

For the TAU condition, more consultations with a psychiatrist and more days in a day-time treatment program in a psychiatric hospital predicted worse treatment outcomes. This could mean that patients' symptomatology and patients' general functioning is too severe to be able to profit from TAU. Furthermore, to our knowledge, there are no international studies regarding psychotherapy of depression, indicating country as a relevant predictor of outcome.

Healthcare utilization within the four months prior starting treatment was found to be a prescriptive predictor in both conditions. Healthcare uptake may be a proxy for a higher somatic or mental burden and/or may represent a more severe symptomatology of depression. In previous studies, more complex cases (e.g., with chronic symptoms and psychiatric comorbidities) or more severe depressive symptomatology predicted a worse therapy outcome [29,38,79–81]. Interestingly, more hospital admissions only predicted worse treatment outcomes in the blended treatment condition. A possible interpretation of this finding is the fact that the online modules in the blended treatment protocol are highly standardized to target depressive symptomatology. As a result, they may have not sufficiently addressed comorbid symptoms. Somatic comorbidities in patients with depression are not a scarcity and have an influence on individual treatment response and illness course, because they can complicate treatment [81]. Furthermore, the number of hospital admissions may also be a proxy for case complexity and higher mental burden, which in turn may have a negative impact on treatment outcome.

This study's results demonstrate that BMA makes it possible to use a limited set of baseline variables to predict treatment outcome. This is in line with a recent study by Bremer and colleagues [42] that showed the feasibility of providing personalized treatment recommendations at baseline regarding clinical and cost-effectiveness using a subsample of the current study by evaluating various machine learning techniques. Moreover, the present study showed that despite sharing the same diagnosis, patients might benefit more from different treatments. The current study found a PAI of 2.33, indicating that patients could have a PHQ-9 score at 12 weeks that is, on average, more than two points lower if they receive their model-determined optimal treatment in comparison to the suboptimal treatment. This value is in the range of other studies that have found PAIs ranging from 1.35 [38] up to 8.9 [40]. Importantly, for almost one-third (29%) of the patients in the present study, a substantial difference was predicted between the two treatment modalities as the individual PAI was 5 or greater. This result is in line with increasing evidence suggesting that differential treatment responses are not rare and might play an important role for an individual patient and the health care system [30].

The current study has several limitations. First of all, the relatively small sample size did not allow us to build and test the models in separate samples. Using the same sample for testing and building the

model might lead to a potential risk of overconfidence. Nevertheless, if studies are designed to develop and validate prescriptive prediction scores that can be tested in future hypothesis-driven confirmatory studies, a smaller sample size might be legitimate [82]. Secondly, the results are based solely on self-reports, and future studies should also include observer ratings. Third, the restricted set of baseline measures is another limitation. Constructs such as personality traits or the familiarity with computers have not been assessed but may have influenced engagement with the online component. Relatedly, people with a low socioeconomic status or senior citizens may not have been well represented in the present study sample. Such groups may not have the opportunity to benefit from the blended treatment, because they may not have access to a computer or a smartphone and/or lack the knowledge to use them. As a consequence, the restricted sample in the present study limits the generalizability of the results. Furthermore, the current study predicts treatment outcome after 12 weeks. Future studies should predict long-term treatment outcome [83]. Finally, we have followed a data-driven approach instead of a theory-driven approach. Although the two methods should be considered complementary [84], a disadvantage of data-driven research is that it is not experiential, and relying on the data alone might not capture the whole picture. Relatedly, the predictors found in the current study need to be validated and replicated in future hypothesis-driven studies.

In spite of the limitations above, the current study is promising to contribute to the further understanding of treatment for depression, because it investigates implications for the use of the blended treatment for patients with depression. Clinical practice should consider factors found to play a role in the treatment and processes of change to provide the optimal treatment for each individual. For example, the quality of life should be taken into account, as these patients may need a more intense treatment protocol that integrates face-to-face interventions with web-based technologies. This interpretation is in line with the notion that more severely depressed patients see the availability of an online program between face-to-face sessions as an advantage of the blended treatment [85]. Furthermore, healthcare utilization should be evaluated prior to treatment selection, because it can give valuable information about the patients' needs, treatment history, and course of illness. In addition, the predictors found to be important in this study and in previous studies could be taken into account to make an informed treatment recommendation in clinical practice. However, future studies with larger samples and more advanced techniques are necessary to validate the current findings, and the identified predictors have to be tested within clinical routine treatment settings. Moreover, prospective studies need to integrate the PAI in the diagnostics process at the beginning of a treatment.

5. Conclusions

To conclude, with the first aim of the study, two prognostic predictors, namely, pretreatment symptomatology and treatment expectancy, were found. Furthermore, several prescriptive predictors were found, predicting the treatment outcome respective of each of the two conditions. Some of our findings are in line with previous research, but other variables, such as baseline healthcare utilization, have not been investigated in this context. The interpretations regarding the prognostic and prescriptive predictors need to be tested empirically, because they are somewhat speculative. Furthermore, this study showed an advantage of model-determined treatment allocation to the TAU or blended treatment, as one-third of the participants had a PAI larger than 5, which means they would have improved significantly if they had received their "optimal" treatment. Although the results need to be validated in future hypothesis-driven studies, the predictors found to be important in the current study should be taken into account to make an informed treatment recommendation in clinical practice.

Supplementary Materials: The following are available online at http://www.mdpi.com/2077-0383/9/2/490/s1: Appendix 1: Bayesian model averaging (BMA) results based on the best 30,000 models in the treatment as usual (TAU) condition, Appendix 2: BMA results based on the best 30,000 models in the blended treatment condition.

Author Contributions: N.F. analyzed the data and wrote the manuscript under the supervision of T.B. All authors critically revised the manuscript and contributed substantially to this work. All authors have read and agreed to the published version of the manuscript.

Funding: This research received no external funding.

Conflicts of Interest: The authors declare no conflict of interest.

References

1. World Health Organization. Depression. 2018. Available online: https://www.who.int/news-room/fact-sheets/detail/depression (accessed on 21 November 2019).
2. World Health Organization. The Global Burden of Disease: 2004 Update. 2008. Available online: https://www.who.int/healthinfo/global_burden_disease/2004_report_update/en/ (accessed on 3 October 2019).
3. Kemmeren, L.; Van Schaik, D.J.; Riper, H.; Kleiboer, A.M.; Bosmans, J.E.; Smit, J.H. Effectiveness of blended depression treatment for adults in specialised mental healthcare: Study protocol for a randomised controlled trial. *BMC Psychiatry* **2016**, *16*, 113. [CrossRef] [PubMed]
4. Karasu, T.B.; Gelenberg, A.; Merriam, A.; Wang, P. Treatment of patients with major depressive disorder. In *American Psychiatric Association Practice Guidelines for the Treatment of Psychiatric Disorders Compendium*; American Psychiatric Publishing: Washington, DC, USA, 2000; pp. 413–495.
5. Cuijpers, P. Psychotherapies for adult depression: Recent developments. *Curr. Opin. Psychiatry* **2015**, *28*, 24–29. [CrossRef] [PubMed]
6. Carlbring, P.; Andersson, G.; Cuijpers, P.; Riper, H.; Hedman-Lagerlöf, E. Internet-based vs. face-to-face cognitive behavior therapy for psychiatric and somatic disorders: An updated systematic review and meta-analysis. *Cognit. Behav. Ther.* **2018**, *47*, 1–18. [CrossRef]
7. Arnberg, F.K.; Linton, S.J.; Hultcrantz, M.; Heintz, E.; Jonsson, U. Internet-delivered psychological treatments for mood and anxiety disorders: A systematic review of their efficacy, safety, and cost-effectiveness. *PLoS ONE* **2014**, *9*, e98118. [CrossRef]
8. Gerhards, S.; De Graaf, L.; Jacobs, L.; Severens, J.; Huibers, M.; Arntz, A.; Riper, H.; Widdershoven, G.; Metsemakers, J.F.M.; Evers, S.M.A.A. Economic evaluation of online computerised cognitive–behavioural therapy without support for depression in primary care: Randomised trial. *Br. J. Psychiatry* **2010**, *196*, 310–318. [CrossRef]
9. Richards, D.; Richardson, T. Computer-based psychological treatments for depression: A systematic review and meta-analysis. *Clin. Psychol. Rev.* **2012**, *32*, 329–342. [CrossRef]
10. Krieger, T.; Meyer, B.; Sude, K.; Urech, A.; Maercker, A.; Berger, T. Evaluating an e-mental health program ("deprexis") as adjunctive treatment tool in psychotherapy for depression: Design of a pragmatic randomized controlled trial. *BMC Psychiatry* **2014**, *14*, 285. [CrossRef]
11. Hickie, I.B.; Davenport, T.A.; Luscombe, G.M.; Moore, M.; Griffiths, K.M.; Christensen, H. Practitioner-supported delivery of internet-based cognitive behaviour therapy: Evaluation of the feasibility of conducting a cluster randomised trial. *Med. J. Aust.* **2010**, *192*, S31–S35. [CrossRef]
12. Høifødt, R.S.; Lillevoll, K.R.; Griffiths, K.M.; Wilsgaard, T.; Eisenmann, M.; Waterloo, K.; Kolstrup, N. The clinical effectiveness of web-based cognitive behavioral therapy with face-to-face therapist support for depressed primary care patients: Randomized controlled trial. *J. Med. Int. Res.* **2013**, *15*, e153.
13. Kessler, D.; Lewis, G.; Kaur, S.; Wiles, N.; King, M.; Weich, S.; Sharp, D.J.; Araya, R.; Hollinghurst, S.; Peters, T.J. Therapist-delivered Internet psychotherapy for depression in primary care: A randomised controlled trial. *Lancet* **2009**, *374*, 628–634. [CrossRef]
14. Kooistra, L.C.; Wiersma, J.E.; Ruwaard, J.; van Oppen, P.; Smit, F.; Lokkerbol, J.; Cuijpers, P.; Riper, H. Blended vs. face-to-face cognitive behavioural treatment for major depression in specialized mental health care: Study protocol of a randomized controlled cost-effectiveness trial. *BMC Psychiatry* **2014**, *14*, 290. [CrossRef]
15. Robertson, L.; Smith, M.; Castle, D.; Tannenbaum, D. Using the Internet to enhance the treatment of depression. *Aust. Psychiatry* **2006**, *14*, 413–417. [CrossRef]
16. Berger, T.; Krieger, T.; Sude, K.; Meyer, B.; Maercker, A. Evaluating an e-mental health program ("deprexis") as adjunctive treatment tool in psychotherapy for depression: Results of a pragmatic randomized controlled trial. *J. Affect. Disord.* **2018**, *227*, 455–462. [CrossRef] [PubMed]
17. Thase, M.E.; Wright, J.H.; Eells, T.D.; Barrett, M.S.; Wisniewski, S.R.; Balasubramani, G.K.; McCrone, P.; Brown, G.K. Improving the efficiency of psychotherapy for depression: Computer-assisted versus standard CBT. *Am. J. Psychiatry* **2017**, *175*, 242–250. [CrossRef] [PubMed]

18. Zwerenz, R.; Becker, J.; Knickenberg, R.J.; Siepmann, M.; Hagen, K.; Beutel, M.E. Online Self-Help as an Add-On to Inpatient Psychotherapy: Efficacy of a New Blended Treatment Approach. *Psychother. Psychosom.* **2017**, *86*, 341–350. [CrossRef] [PubMed]
19. Erbe, D.; Eichert, H.-C.; Riper, H.; Ebert, D.D. Blending face-to-face and internet-based interventions for the treatment of mental disorders in adults: Systematic review. *J. Med. Int. Res.* **2017**, *19*, e306. [CrossRef] [PubMed]
20. Wright, J.H.; Wright, A.S.; Albano, A.M.; Basco, M.R.; Goldsmith, L.J.; Raffield, T.; Otto, M.W. Computer-assisted cognitive therapy for depression: Maintaining efficacy while reducing therapist time. *Am. J. Psychiatry* **2005**, *162*, 1158–1164. [CrossRef]
21. Clough, B.A.; Casey, L.M. Technological adjuncts to increase adherence to therapy: A review. *Clin. Psychol. Rev.* **2011**, *31*, 697–710. [CrossRef]
22. Riper, H.; Van Ballegooijen, W.; Kooistra, L.; De Wit, J.; Donker, T. *Preventie & eMental-Health-Prevention & eMental-Health*; Vrije Universiteit Commissioned by ZonMw: Amsterdam, The Netherlands, 2013.
23. Van der Vaart, R.; Witting, M.; Riper, H.; Kooistra, L.; Bohlmeijer, E.T.; van Gemert-Pijnen, L.J. Blending online therapy into regular face-to-face therapy for depression: Content, ratio and preconditions according to patients and therapists using a Delphi study. *BMC Psychiatry* **2014**, *14*, 355. [CrossRef]
24. Wentzel, J.; van der Vaart, R.; Bohlmeijer, E.T.; van Gemert-Pijnen, J.E. Mixing online and face-to-face therapy: How to benefit from blended care in mental health care. *JMIR Mental Health* **2016**, *3*, e9. [CrossRef]
25. Ruwaard, J.; Kok, R. Wild West eHealth: Time to hold our horses? *Eur. Health Psychol.* **2015**, *17*, 45–49.
26. Zilcha-Mano, S. Major developments in methods addressing for whom psychotherapy may work and why. *Psychother. Res.* **2018**, *29*, 693–708. [CrossRef] [PubMed]
27. Kazdin, A.E. Evidence-based treatment and practice: New opportunities to bridge clinical research and practice, enhance the knowledge base, and improve patient care. *Am. Psychol.* **2008**, *63*, 146. [CrossRef] [PubMed]
28. Cuijpers, P.; Van Straten, A.; Bohlmeijer, E.; Hollon, S.D.; Andersson, G. The effects of psychotherapy for adult depression are overestimated: A meta-analysis of study quality and effect size. *Psychol. Med.* **2010**, *40*, 211–223. [CrossRef]
29. Fournier, J.C.; DeRubeis, R.J.; Shelton, R.C.; Hollon, S.D.; Amsterdam, J.D.; Gallop, R. Prediction of response to medication and cognitive therapy in the treatment of moderate to severe depression. *J. Consult. Clin. Psychol.* **2009**, *77*, 775. [CrossRef]
30. Cohen, Z.D.; DeRubeis, R.J. Treatment selection in depression. *Ann. Rev. Clin. Psychol.* **2018**, *14*, 209–236. [CrossRef]
31. Fisher, A.J.; Boswell, J.F. Enhancing the personalization of psychotherapy with dynamic assessment and modeling. *Assessment* **2016**, *23*, 496–506. [CrossRef]
32. Hollon, S.D.; Cohne, Z.D.; Singla, D.R.; Andrews, P. Recent Developments in the Treatment of Depression. *Behav. Ther.* **2019**, *50*, 257–269. [CrossRef]
33. Hamburg, M.A.; Collins, F.S. The path to personalized medicine. *N. Engl. J. Med.* **2010**, *363*, 301–304. [CrossRef]
34. Van Bronswijk, S.C.; Lemmens, L.H.; Keefe, J.R.; Huibers, M.J.; DeRubeis, R.J.; Peeters, F.P. A prognostic index for long-term outcome after successful acute phase cognitive therapy and interpersonal psychotherapy for major depressive disorder. *Depress. Anxiety* **2018**, *36*, 252–261. [CrossRef]
35. Becker, D.; van Breda, W.; Funk, B.; Hoogendoorn, M.; Ruwaard, J.; Riper, H. Predictive modeling in e-mental health: A common language framework. *Internet Interv.* **2018**, *12*, 57–67. [CrossRef] [PubMed]
36. DeRubeis, R.J.; Cohen, Z.D.; Forand, N.R.; Fournier, J.C.; Gelfand, L.A.; Lorenzo-Luaces, L. The Personalized Advantage Index: Translating research on prediction into individualized treatment recommendations. A demonstration. *PLoS ONE* **2014**, *9*, e83875. [CrossRef] [PubMed]
37. Cohen, Z.D.; Kim, T.; Van, H.; Dekker, J.; Driessen, E. Recommending Cognitive-Behavioral Versus Psychodynamic Therapy for Mild to Moderate Adult Depression. *Psychother. Res.* **2017**, *30*, 137–150. [CrossRef] [PubMed]
38. Friedl, N.; Berger, T.; Krieger, T.; Caspar, F.; Grosse Holtforth, M. Using the Personalized Advantage Index for individual treatment allocation to cognitive behavioral therapy (CBT) or a CBT with integrated exposure and emotion-focused elements (CBT-EE). *Psychother. Res.* **2019**. [CrossRef]

39. DeRubeis, R.J.; Hollon, S.D.; Amsterdam, J.D.; Shelton, R.C.; Young, P.R.; Salomon, R.M.; O'Reardon, J.P.; Lovett, M.L.; Gladis, M.M.; Brown, L.L. Cognitive therapy vs. medications in the treatment of moderate to severe depression. *Arch. Gen. Psychiatry* **2005**, *62*, 409–416. [CrossRef]
40. Huibers, M.J.; Cohen, Z.D.; Lemmens, L.H.; Arntz, A.; Peeters, F.P.; Cuijpers, P.; DeRubeis, R.J. Predicting optimal outcomes in cognitive therapy or interpersonal psychotherapy for depressed individuals using the personalized advantage index approach. *PLoS ONE* **2015**, *10*, e0140771. [CrossRef]
41. Van Breda, W.; Bremer, V.; Becker, D.; Hoogendoorn, M.; Funk, B.; Ruwaard, J.; Riper, H. Predicting therapy success for treatment as usual and blended treatment in the domain of depression. *Internet Interv.* **2018**, *12*, 100–104. [CrossRef]
42. Bremer, V.; Becker, D.; Kolovos, S.; Funk, B.; Van Breda, W.; Hoogendoorn, M.; Riper, H. Predicting therapy success and costs for personalized treatment recommendations using baseline characteristics: Data-driven analysis. *J. Med. Internet Res.* **2018**, *20*, e10275. [CrossRef]
43. Kleiboer, A.; Smit, J.; Bosmans, J.; Ruwaard, J.; Andersson, G.; Topooco, N.; Berger, T.; Krieger, T.; Botella, C.; Banos, R. European COMPARative Effectiveness research on blended Depression treatment versus treatment-as-usual (E-COMPARED): Study protocol for a randomized controlled, non-inferiority trial in eight European countries. *Trials* **2016**, *17*, 387. [CrossRef]
44. Sheehan, D.V.; Lecrubier, Y.; Sheehan, K.H.; Amorim, P.; Janavs, J.; Weiller, E.; Hergueta, T.; Baker, R.; Dunbar, G.C. The Mini-International Neuropsychiatric Interview (MINI): The development and validation of a structured diagnostic psychiatric interview for DSM-IV and ICD-10. *J. Clin. Psychiatry* **1998**, *59*, 22–33.
45. Kroenke, K.; Spitzer, R.L.; Williams, J.B. The PHQ-9: Validity of a brief depression severity measure. *J. Gen. Intern. Med.* **2001**, *16*, 606–613. [CrossRef] [PubMed]
46. Meyer, B.; Berger, T.; Caspar, F.; Beevers, C.G.; Andersson, G.; Weiss, M. Effectiveness of a Novel Integrative Online Treatment for Depression (Deprexis): Randomized Controlled Trial. *J. Med. Internet Res.* **2009**, *11*, e15. [CrossRef] [PubMed]
47. Mathiasen, K.; Andersen, T.E.; Riper, H.; Kleiboer, A.A.; Roessler, K.K. Blended CBT versus face-to-face CBT: A randomised non-inferiority trial. *BMC Psychiatry* **2016**, *16*, 432. [CrossRef] [PubMed]
48. Kroenke, K. Enhancing the clinical utility of depression screening. *CMAJ Can. Med. Assoc. J.* **2012**, *184*, 281–282. [CrossRef] [PubMed]
49. Kroenke, K.; Spitzer, R.L. The PHQ-9: A new depression diagnostic and severity measure. *Psychiatr. Ann.* **2002**, *32*, 509–515. [CrossRef]
50. Manea, L.; Gilbody, S.; McMillan, D. Optimal cut-off score for diagnosing depression with the Patient Health Questionnaire (PHQ-9): A meta-analysis. *Can. Med. Assoc. J.* **2012**, *184*, E191–E196. [CrossRef]
51. EuroQol. EuroQol—A new facility for the measurement of health-related quality of life. *Health Policy* **1990**, *16*, 199–208.
52. Bouwmans, C.; De Jong, K.; Timman, R.; Zijlstra-Vlasveld, M.; Van der Feltz-Cornelis, C.; Tan, S.S.; Hakkaart-van Roijen, L. Feasibility, reliability and validity of a questionnaire on healthcare consumption and productivity loss in patients with a psychiatric disorder (TiC-P). *BMC Health Serv. Res.* **2013**, *13*, 217. [CrossRef] [PubMed]
53. Devilly, G.J.; Borkovec, T.D. Psychometric properties of the credibility/expectancy questionnaire. *J. Behav. Ther. Exp. Psychiatry* **2000**, *31*, 73–86. [CrossRef]
54. Stekhoven, D.J. *Missforest: Nonparametric Missing Value Imputation Using Random Forest*; R Package Version, 1; Astrophysics Source Code Library: Leicester, UK, 2013.
55. Stekhoven, D.J.; Buhlmann, P. MissForest: Non-parametric missing value imputation for mixed-type data. *Bioinformatics* **2012**, *28*, 112–118. [CrossRef]
56. Waljee, A.K.; Mukherjee, A.; Singal, A.G.; Zhang, Y.; Warren, J.; Balis, U.; Marrero, J.; Zhu, J.; Higgins, P.D. Comparison of imputation methods for missing laboratory data in medicine. *BMJ Open* **2013**, *3*, e002847. [CrossRef]
57. Peduzzi, P.; Concato, J.; Feinstein, A.R.; Holford, T.R. Importance of events per independent variable in proportional hazards regression analysis II. Accuracy and precision of regression estimates. *J. Clin. Epidemiol.* **1995**, *48*, 1503–1510. [CrossRef]
58. Vittinghoff, E.; McCulloch, C.E. Relaxing the rule of ten events per variable in logistic and Cox regression. *Am. J. Epidemiol.* **2007**, *165*, 710–718. [CrossRef] [PubMed]

59. Raftery, A.E.; Madigan, D.; Hoeting, J.A. Bayesian model averaging for linear regression models. *J. Am. Stat. Assoc.* **1997**, *92*, 179–191. [CrossRef]
60. Stock, E.M.; Kimbrel, N.A.; Meyer, E.C.; Copeland, L.A.; Monte, R ; Zeber, J.E.; Gulliver, S.B.; Morissette, S.B. A Bayesian model averaging approach to examining changes in quality of life among returning Iraq and Afghanistan Veterans. *Int. J. Methods Psychiatry Res.* **2014**, *23*, 345–358. [CrossRef] [PubMed]
61. Babyak, M.A. What you see may not be what you get: A brief, nontechnical introduction to overfitting in regression-type models. *Psychosom. Med.* **2004**, *66*, 411–421.
62. Fragoso, T.M.; Bertoli, W.; Louzada, F. Bayesian model averaging: A systematic review and conceptual classification. *Int. Stat. Rev.* **2018**, *86*, 1–28. [CrossRef]
63. Fernandez, C.; Ley, E.; Steel, M.F. Benchmark priors for Bayesian model averaging. *J. Econom.* **2001**, *100*, 381–427. [CrossRef]
64. Fernandez, C.; Ley, E.; Steel, M.F. Model uncertainty in cross-country growth regressions. *J. Appl. Econom.* **2001**, *16*, 563–576. [CrossRef]
65. Ley, E.; Steel, M.F.J. On the effect of prior assumptions in Bayesian model averaging with applications to growth regression. *J. Appl. Econom.* **2009**, *24*, 651–674. [CrossRef]
66. Steel, M.F. Bayesian model averaging and forecasting. *Bull. Inflat Macroecon. Anal.* **2011**, *200*, 30–41.
67. Clyde, M.A. BAS: Bayesian Variable Selection and Model Averaging using Bayesian. In *Adaptive Sampling*; 2018; R Package Version 1.5.3; Available online: https://cran.r-project.org/web/packages/BAS/BAS.pdf (accessed on 15 September 2019).
68. Clyde, M.A.; Ghosh, J.; Littman, M.L. Bayesian adaptive sampling for variable selection and model averaging. *J. Comput. Gr. Stat.* **2011**, *20*, 80–101. [CrossRef]
69. Efron, B.; Gong, G. A leisurely look at the bootstrap, the jackknife, and cross-validation. *Am. Stat.* **1983**, *37*, 36–48.
70. Deisenhofer, A.K.; Delgadillo, J.; Rubel, J.A.; Böhnke, J.R.; Zimmermann, D.; Schwartz, B.; Lutz, W. Individual treatment selection for patients with posttraumatic stress disorder. *Depress. Anxiety* **2018**, *35*, 541–550. [CrossRef]
71. Lowe, B.; Unutzer, J.; Callahan, C.M.; Perkins, A.J.; Kroenke, K. Monitoring depression treatment outcomes with the patient health questionnaire-9. *Med. Care* **2004**, *42*, 1194–1201.
72. Dinga, R.; Marquand, A.F.; Veltman, D.J.; Beekman, A.T.F.; Schoevers, R.A.; van Hemert, A.M.; Penninx, B.; Schmaal, L. Predicting the naturalistic course of depression from a wide range of clinical, psychological, and biological data: A machine learning approach. *Transl. Psychiatry* **2018**, *8*, 241. [CrossRef]
73. Hamilton, K.E.; Dobson, K.S. Cognitive therapy of depression: Pretreatment patient predictors of outcome. *Clin. Psychol. Rev.* **2002**, *22*, 875–893. [CrossRef]
74. Constantino, M.J.; Arnkoff, D.B.; Glass, C.R.; Ametrano, R.M.; Smith, J.Z. Expectations. *J. Clin. Psychol.* **2011**, *67*, 184–192. [CrossRef]
75. Greenberg, R.P.; Constantino, M.J.; Bruce, N. Are patient expectations still relevant for psychotherapy process and outcome? *Clin. Psychol. Rev.* **2006**, *26*, 657–678. [CrossRef]
76. Spek, V.; Nyklíček, I.; Cuijpers, P.; Pop, V. Predictors of outcome of group and internet-based cognitive behavior therapy. *J. Affect. Disord.* **2008**, *105*, 137–145. [CrossRef]
77. Andersson, G.; Hedman, E. Effectiveness of guided internet-based cognitive behavior therapy in regular clinical settings. *Verhaltenstherapie* **2013**, *23*, 140–148. [CrossRef]
78. Bower, P.; Kontopantelis, E.; Sutton, A.; Kendrick, T.; Richards, D.A.; Gillbody, S.; Knowles, S.; Cuijpers, P.; Andersson, G.; Christensen, H.; et al. Influence of initial severity of depression on effectiveness of low intensity interventions: Meta-analysis of individual patient data. *BMJ (Clin. Res.)* **2013**, *346*, f540. [CrossRef]
79. Thase, M.E.; Reynolds, C.F.; Frank, E.; Simons, A.D. Response to cognitive-behavioral therapy in chronic depression. *J. Psychother. Pract. Res.* **1994**, *3*, 304–314.
80. Blom, M.B.; Spinhoven, P.; Hoffman, T.; Jonker, K.; Hoencamp, E.; Haffmans, P.J.; van Dyck, R. Severity and duration of depression, not personality factors, predict short term outcome in the treatment of major depression. *J. Affect. Disord.* **2007**, *104*, 119–126. [CrossRef]
81. Delgadillo, J.; Huey, D.; Bennett, H.; McMillan, D. Case complexity as a guide for psychological treatment selection. *J. Consult. Clin. Psychol.* **2017**, *85*, 835–853. [CrossRef]

82. Luedtke, A.; Sadikova, E.; Kessler, R.C. Sample Size Requirements for Multivariate Models to Predict Between-Patient Differences in Best Treatments of Major Depressive Disorder. *Clin. Psychol. Sci.* **2019**, *7*, 445–461. [CrossRef]
83. Van Bronswijk, S.C.; DeRubeis, R.J.; Lemmens, L.H.; Peeters, F.P.; Keefe, J.R.; Cohen, Z.D.; Huibers, M. Precision medicine for long-term depression outcomes using the Personalized Advantage Index approach: Cognitive therapy or interpersonal psychotherapy? *Psychol. Med.* **2019**, 1–11. [CrossRef]
84. Gillan, C.M.; Whelan, D.R. What big data can do for treatment in psychiatry. *Curr. Opin. Behav. Sci.* **2017**, *18*, 34–42. [CrossRef]
85. Urech, A.; Krieger, T.; Möseneder, L.; Biaggi, A.; Vincent, A.; Poppe, C.; Meyer, B.; Riper, H.; Berger, T. A patient post hoc perspective on advantages and disadvantages of blended cognitive behaviour therapy for depression: A qualitative content analysis. *Psychother. Res.* **2019**, *29*, 986–998. [CrossRef]

Journal of
Clinical Medicine

MDPI

Article

ZIEL: Internet-Based Self-Help for Adjustment Problems: Results of a Randomized Controlled Trial

Christian Moser [1,*], Rahel Bachem [2], Thomas Berger [1] and Andreas Maercker [2]

1 Clinical Psychology and Psychotherapy, University of Bern, 3012 Bern, Switzerland; thomas.berger@psy.unibe.ch

2 Psychopathology and Clinical Intervention, University of Zürich, 8050 Zürich, Switzerland; rahel.bachem@gmail.com (R.B.); maercker@psychologie.uzh.ch (A.M.)

* Correspondence: christian.moser@psy.unibe.ch

Received: 28 August 2019; Accepted: 5 October 2019; Published: 11 October 2019

Abstract: Adjustment Disorder (AjD) represents a healthcare paradox. On the one hand, it is one of the most diagnosed mental disorders worldwide. On the other hand, AjD and its possible treatment options remain a severely neglected field of research. In this context, we developed a self-guided online intervention for adjustment problems, named ZIEL, and tested its efficacy. It is based on and extends a bibliotherapeutic treatment approach for symptoms of AjD. In our study, a total of 98 individuals who had experienced a life event in the last two years, were randomly assigned to care as usual (CAU) or an online intervention group (CAU + online intervention). The primary endpoint was AjD symptom severity measured by Adjustment Disorder–New Module 20 (ADNM-20). Secondary endpoints were depressive symptoms, quality of life and other variables such as satisfaction and usability. Both the intervention and the control group improved comparably well regarding the severity of adjustment disorder symptoms post-treatment. However, participants in the intervention group showed significantly fewer depressive symptoms and a significantly higher quality of life (Cohen's d: 0.89 (BDI) and −0.49 (SF-12)). The intervention was well-received by users with an above average usability rating. Overall, the results suggest that the ZIEL intervention has the promise to contribute to the treatment of AjD and reduce symptom burden by means of a scalable low-barrier approach.

Keywords: adjustment disorder; e-mental health; self-guided intervention; disorders specifically related to stress

---

1. Introduction

"It's really wonderful how much resilience there is in human nature," famous Dracula novelist Stoker stated at the end of the 19th century, against the background of his own adverse experiences [1]

However, there are events in the lives of people that can exceed their psychological resilience. Adjustment Disorder (AjD) marks the transition between normal stress response and impairments with clinically relevant severity or duration [2]. Even if the specific nature of this shift is debated, it does exist [3,4]. What is remarkable, however, is the extent to which the state of clinical practice diverges from the research efforts on AjD. On the one hand, it is one of the most diagnosed mental disorders worldwide [5]. On the other hand, research on AjD and its possible treatment remain a severely neglected field of study [6].

One reason for the gap between practice and research is the lack of diagnostic reliability and validity of AjD, in its ICD-10 and DSM-5 sub-threshold conceptualization [7–9]. However, the evidence base for a full-threshold understanding has been increasing. Amongst others, this includes an equal symptom-severity to e.g., major depression, a lowered quality of life and comparably earlier execution of suicidal ideations [10–13]. Consequently, a re-conceptualization of AjD in the ICD-11 was achieved [4].

It is now being recognized as a full-threshold disorder with the core symptoms of preoccupation with the stressor (e.g., constant rumination) and failure to adapt (e.g., concentration problems) [14].

The importance of this change becomes apparent when looking at the current AjD health care situation. A large proportion of diagnosed individuals do not receive treatment at all [15]. The majority that do, receive it in primary health care settings. Here, AjD is just as likely to be treated with pharmacotherapy like other severe mental disorders; the crucial difference being, that there is no evidence base for this practice with AjD [4,16]. As Strain and Friedman recommend, the first-line of treatment for AjD is psychotherapy, where different general approaches like Cognitive Behavioral Therapy, Eye-Movement Desensitization and Reprocessing, Client-centered Psychotherapy and various brief psychological interventions have been tested with varying success [17–20]. Disorder-specific approaches are rare, but they do exist.

Regarding this scarcity of disorder-specific AjD treatment approaches, there have been various new impulses in the context of Internet-based interventions for AjD in recent years. One of the first digital AjD-specific treatments used Virtual Reality elements to enhance a face-to-face intervention. So-called "EMMA's World", proved to be an effective alternative to traditional treatment and led to significant improvements in areas of depression, relaxation and social interactions for participants [21]. A more recent development of the same group, called TAO, is currently being tested [22]. It combines approaches from cognitive-behavioral therapy (CBT) and Positive Psychology for the guided treatment of AjD. Preliminary findings show good results for both user-friendliness and acceptance for participants [23]. A different approach is pursued with BADI (Brief Adjustment Disorder Intervention), a self-guided intervention for AjD [24]. It combines exercises in relaxation, time management, mindfulness and coping with interpersonal difficulties. Results of a randomized controlled trial show a medium effect size of the intervention on adjustment disorder symptoms [24]. Lastly, there is a new guided online intervention for chronic stress, that explicitly includes AjD. It uses a larger catalog of contemporary CBT techniques, e.g., exposure, sleep management and behavioral activation. A first trial showed moderate to large improvements in terms of perceived stress, as well as in functional impairment and work ability [24].

From a client's point of view, internet-based interventions offer significant advantages, some of which make AjD uniquely suited for this approach [25,26]. First, there is the potential for optimal timing of the intervention. In principle, online interventions could be made available immediately after the occurrence of an adverse life event, for example, via smartphone. This also eliminates the stigma, that would typically be associated with both a strong reaction to a stressor and a visit of a therapist, and usually prevents many individuals from utilizing available help [27]. Finally, the main advantage of self-guided interventions, in particular, is their enormous scalability. It allows not just for consistent availability of services but also ensures economic viability. Both the cost of distribution and the marginal costs added by each new user, converge towards zero with larger numbers of participants.

At the same time, digitalization also opens new possibilities for researchers and practitioners. A central idea is an iterative and incremental approach, as it is part for example, of the agile software development framework [28]. Instead of strictly sequential production, one assumes continuous development of an intervention, driven by constant learning. This has various advantages. Firstly, it allows for rapid iterations of just specific parts of either the content or technology. Scope and functionality can be efficiently expanded based on momentary resources and needs [26]. Secondly, the software allows for detailed analytics of use. With little additional effort, different functionalities or variants of modules can be tested in direct comparison [29]. Thirdly, the translational lag with the transfer of current research findings into clinical practice is significantly shorter than with traditional approaches [30]. Altogether, this bears the potential to significantly improve the quality and availability of care for individuals in need on a long-term basis.

These considerations form the basis of this study and its two objectives: Firstly, the development of a sustainable self-guided intervention for AjD called "Back to your own life (German acronym: ZIEL)." Secondly, to test the efficacy of this intervention, compared to a care as usual control group

(CAU). We hypothesized that the active treatment condition would be superior to CAU on measures of AjD symptom severity and that effects would be stable in the three-month follow-up. The goal is to contribute and to expand the growing efforts in the field of AjD research and care.

2. Experimental Section

2.1. Study Design

This randomized controlled trial (RCT) compared an immediate intervention group with a CAU-only control group. The program was only accessible during the intervention stage. The participants of the control group got their access after the four-week post-assessment. The immediate intervention group was followed up until three months after randomization to examine the stability of potential gains. The trial was registered with Clinicaltrials.gov and was approved by the Ethics Committee of the School of Arts and Science at the University of Zürich, Switzerland (1 February 2016) [31].

2.2. Recruitment

We recruited individuals from the general population from January 2018 until March 2019. For this purpose, we used a study recruitment web page, which was advertised on various websites, forums, and social media. Additionally, we advertised the study at various psychiatric hospitals around Switzerland. The study web page presented general information about adjustment problems and AjD, an outline of the study, a link to 24 h emergency phone numbers, and a registration form.

Individuals who registered received detailed information about the study via e-mail. Individuals who signed informed consent were asked to complete online self-report questionnaires. Based on the answers, the eligibility criteria were assessed. For inclusion, the following criteria had to be met: Minimum age of 18 years, the existence of an emergency address and a life event between two weeks and two years before the participation that still negatively impacts their lives. The latter recorded by means of the Adjustment Disorder-New Module 20 (ADNM-20) stressor list.

The following criteria led to exclusion: Moderate or severe depressive symptoms (BDI > 18), suicidality (BDI suicidality item > 1), a diagnosis of psychotic, bipolar or other serious mental or physical disorders requiring immediate treatment. Individuals who did not meet the criteria were referred to adequate services and had the opportunity to access the intervention outside of the study.

2.3. Enrollment

A flowchart of the enrollment sequence is depicted in Figure 1. A total of 421 individuals signed up on the recruitment site, 315 gave informed consent and completed the baseline questionnaires. Out of those, 217 had to be excluded based on the inclusion and exclusion criteria. The remaining 98 participants were randomly assigned to one of the two trial conditions: the CAU plus internet intervention condition or the CAU control condition. Randomization was carried out by an independent researcher at the University of Bern. The independent researcher used anonymized numbers for the allocation, via a pre-produced 1:1 ratio, random sequence [32]. The allocation list was concealed from the investigators and participants. After the randomization, the participants received an email regarding their allocation.

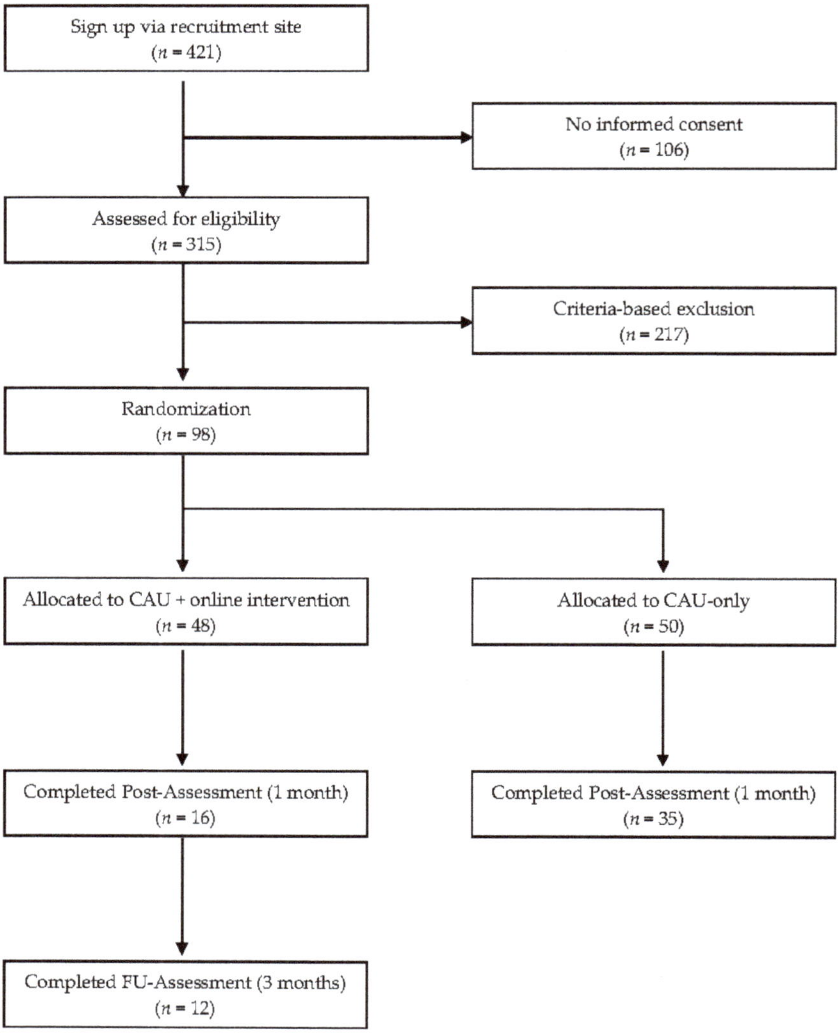

Figure 1. Participant flow.

2.4. Online Intervention

2.4.1. Platform

Technologically, we wanted to create the conditions for continuous in-house intervention-development. A platform should enable us to efficiently adapt to advancements in research and on the end-user side. Consequently, we have aimed to implement powerful open source components whenever possible. One example would be the front-end toolkit Bootstrap that we used for mobile-first interface design [33]. In addition to high quality, the use of popular tools provides good accessibility for potential follow-up projects.

Another aim that guided development was a good user experience (UX) throughout the study. One instance of how this goal manifests itself, is the so called reduction of friction. In the context of UX, this is understood to mean that the intervention is used with as little disruption and frustration as possible to prevent users from abandoning their tasks at hand. An example of this would be the registration, as the first entry point to the study. Contrary to a common multi-step procedure, ZIEL-users could enter the registration-process with just one click of a button.

2.4.2. Intervention

The intervention is based on a manual by Bachem and Maercker [34]. This manual is aimed at AjD for burglary victims and has already been successfully tested in a paper-based version [35]. Based on the theoretical model of AjD for the ICD-11, it integrates evidence-based techniques from the areas of post-traumatic stress disorder, anxiety disorders and depression [36]. The intervention is to be carried out over 4 weeks, whereby the content can be freely chosen by the users according to their current needs or symptoms.

In the first part, users are introduced to the concept of AjD and guided to assess their current symptom burden. Building on this, they get support in deciding whether the intervention is appropriate or whether it is better to make use of traditional support services. This is followed by a second part with self-help exercises, modelled along symptoms or symptom clusters as typically experienced by those affected.

In the first section on sense of self, the stress response and previous coping strategies are examined in more detail, also in light of existing risk and protective factors. In the second section on coping, a series of cognitive strategies are introduced in order to learn how to deal better with presenting burdens. These include techniques such as stopping thoughts from ruminating, as well as correcting cognitive biases (i.e., addressing preoccupations). In the third section on activation, the user deals primarily with the utilization of personal resources at various levels. This includes functional goal setting as well as e.g., the initiation of physical activities (i.e., addressing failure to adapt symptoms). Lastly, the section on recovery covers how activity and rest phases can best be kept in balance in the future, as well as a number of relaxation techniques. Table 1 depicts the details of the content sections.

Table 1. Section overview.

Section 1: Introduction	Psychoeducation; learning to evaluate the psychological burden caused by a life event; deciding about the adequacy of the intervention.
Section 2: Sense of self	Analyzing the individual adjustment reaction; learning about risk and protective factors; inspecting individual former coping strategies.
Section 3: Coping	Recognizing and correcting cognitive biases; writing a narrative exposure exercise; managing anxiety and rumination.
Section 4: Activation	Physical exercising; setting realistic positive goals; regaining positive experiences; evaluating milestones of the personal history.
Section 5: Recovery	Learning to balance activity and relaxation; getting to know various approaches to relaxation; improving sleep and imaginative techniques.

The preservation of a self-directed approach resulted from the perspective of a possible scalable implementation in a standard care setting. After a negative life event, there is a time window of about one month in which a possible development of AjD takes place [14]. In order to support affected people to a relevant extent on such short notice, a reliance on skilled workforce would not be feasible regarding availability and organization. Closely related is the decision in favor of a completely anonymous and automated usage scenario. Social barriers to timely care should be eliminated as far as possible. Finally, the content was re-written agnostic of a specific stressor, restructured into shorter text-sections and additionally made available as audio versions. Figure A1 shows illustrative screenshots of the intervention.

2.5. Outcome Measures

2.5.1. Adjustment Disorder Symptom Severity

The Adjustment Disorder-New Module 20 (ADNM-20) is a self-report questionnaire to track life events and identify adjustment issues. In the first part, it records acute and chronic life events by means of a semi-structured stressor list. In the second part, the AjD core symptoms of preoccupation and failure to adapt (4 items each) as well as accessory symptoms of avoidance, depressive mood, anxiety and impulse disturbance (12 items) are measured. All 20 items are measured on a 4-point Likert-type scale (1 = *never*, 4 = *often*) [37]. Additionally, a total sum score indicates the overall symptom burden and allows for the identification of high risk for AjD (score above 47.5) [38]. The scale offers satisfactory psychometric properties as shown in previous studies [36,37]. The internal consistency of the ADNM-20 in the present study was good for the sum score (Cronbach's α 0.85), and acceptable for the subscales preoccupations (Cronbach's α 0.78), failure to adapt (Cronbach's α 0.73) and good for the accessory symptoms (Cronbach's α 0.83).

2.5.2. General Psychopathology

The Brief Symptom Inventory, Short Form (BSI-18) is a self-report questionnaire to assess general psychological distress. Syndromes of somatization, depression, and anxiety are measured by 18 items on a 5-point Likert-type scale (0 = not at all, 4 = very strong) [39]. The BSI-18 exhibits robust psychometric qualities in previous studies [38]. In the present study, Cronbach's α was 0.82.

2.5.3. Depressive Symptoms

The Beck Depression Inventory (BDI) is a self-report questionnaire to assess depressive symptoms. Each of the 21 items is rated on a 4-point Likert-type scale (0 = not at all, 3 = very strong) [40]. The BDI offers sufficient psychometrics properties [41]. In the present study, Cronbach's α was 0.77.

2.5.4. Quality of Life

The Short Form Health Survey–12 (SF-12) is a self-report questionnaire to assess health-related quality of life. Both a physical and a mental health index are measured by 12 items on a 5-point Likert-type scale [42]. The instrument shows robust psychometrics properties [43]. In the present study, Cronbach's α for the mental health subscale was 0.78 and for the physical health subscale, 0.76.

2.5.5. Expectations about Treatment

The Credibility/Expectancy Questionnaire (CEQ) is a self-report questionnaire to assess treatment expectancy and the credibility of its rationale. The subscales of treatment credibility and outcome expectation are measured by six items in total, each on a scale of 1 (not at all) to 9 (very much). The CEQ exhibits robust psychometric qualities [44]. In the present study, Cronbach's α was 0.88.

2.5.6. Usability

The System Usability Scale (SUS) is a self-report questionnaire to assess the usability of a system. Each of the ten items was adapted to the use-case and is measured on a 5-point Likert-type scale (1 = strongly agree, five strongly disagree) [45]. The SUS offers robust psychometric properties [46]. In the present study, Cronbach's α was 0.84.

2.5.7. Adherence

The intervention platform automatically registered various indices of adherence for each anonymized account-ID: Number of logins, individual pageviews, pageviews per login, total and average time spent in the intervention.

2.6. Power Analysis

The power analysis was conducted with G*Power 3 to determine the appropriate sample size for the detection of differences between the two groups [47]. We aimed at the detection of a medium effect size of 0.5, based on previous research by Eimontas et al. [22]. Accordingly, a power analysis showed that with an alpha error level of 0.05 and a power of (1-beta) of 0.80 about 128 individuals would be needed.

2.7. Statistical Analysis

To test group differences in both demographic data and baseline measures, independent sample *t*-tests, respectively χ^2-tests for nominal data variables were used. Differential outcomes at posttreatment were evaluated according to an intention-to-treat principle using a mixed-model repeated-measures analysis of variance with time (pre-post) as a within-group factor and treatment condition as a between-group factor. This approach was favored as it uses all available data of each subject. Missing values are not substituted; rather parameters of missing values are estimated [48]. Within- and between-group effect sizes (Cohen's d) were calculated based on estimated means and the pooled standard deviation from the observed means. Within-group changes in outcome scores from posttreatment to follow-up were analyzed using paired *t*-tests for people who completed the post and the follow-up-assessment in the intervention group only. To test predictions to the outcome, we calculated linear regression models regressing each adherence measure on the 4-week primary outcome (ADNM-20) controlling for baseline scores in the intervention group. Post hoc tests were Bonferroni corrected for multiple comparisons. All analysis was performed in R and the package lme4 [49,50].

3. Results

3.1. Pre-Treatment Evaluation

The conditions in both groups did not differ in terms of AjD symptom burden or demographic characteristics. The incidence of AjD in the intervention group was 71% (n = 34) and 72% in the CAU group (n = 36). Table 2 provides corresponding details for demographic characteristics. Likewise, the perception of credibility and expectancy of the intervention was the same for participants in both conditions ($p > 0.47$).

3.2. Dropout Analysis

Overall, 47 (active, n = 32; CAU, n = 15) participants (48%) did not complete the posttreatment assessment, even though they had been invited three times in weekly intervals via automated email. The difference in response between the two groups is significant ($p < 0.01$). This can likely be attributed to the fact, that the control group did not gain access to the intervention until after completing the post-assessments. Reasons for dropping out remained unknown since there was no way to reach and question the respective users. As for predictors of dropout, there were no significant differences observed in terms of demographics, pre-treatment or post-treatment scores (all *p*s > 0.21) between those who provided data and those who did not.

3.3. Treatment Outcomes

The observed and estimated means for the self-report questionnaires are presented in Table 3. Mixed-model linear regression analysis with group as a fixed factor and time as a repeated factor (pre-post) were conducted for each of the dependent outcome measures.

Table 2. Pre-Treatment Evaluation.

	Intervention Group $n = 48$	CAU-Only Group $n = 50$	Statistic
Mean age, years (SD)	40.54 (13.0)	40.28 (12.8)	$t(96) = 0.10$ $p = 0.92$
Gender n (%)			
Female	40 (83.3)	44 (88.0)	$Chi^2 = 0.44$ $p = 0.51$
Male	8 (16.7)	6 (12.0)	
Marital status, n (%)			
Single	11 (22.9)	10 (20.0)	$Chi^2 = 2.06$ $p = 0.72$
Married	28 (37.5)	24 (48.0)	
Living together	10 (20.8)	11 (22.0)	
Divorced	7 (14.6)	4 (8.0)	
Widowed	2 (4.2)	1 (2.0)	
Number of kids, n (%)			
None	23 (47.9)	27 (54.0)	$Chi^2 = 3.36$ $p = 0.50$
One	7 (14.6)	11 (22.0)	
Two	13 (27.1)	10 (20.0)	
Three	4 (8.3)	1 (2.0)	
More than three	1 (2.1)	1 (2.0)	
Employment, n (%)			
Full-time paid work	13 (27.1)	23 (46.0)	$Chi^2 = 5.60$ $p = 0.35$
Part-time paid work	19 (39.6)	15 (30.0)	
Unemployed	2 (4.2)	2 (4.0)	
At home parent	4 (8.3)	1 (2.0)	
Student	5 (10.4)	3 (6.0)	
Retired	5 (10.4)	6 (12.0)	
Highest education, n (%)			
Compulsory school	1 (2.1)	0 (0.0)	$Chi^2 = 5.06$ $p = 0.17$
Apprenticeship	15 (31.3)	8 (16.0)	
College	5 (10.4)	4 (8.0)	
University	27 (56.3)	38 (76.0)	
Current psychological treatment, n (%)			
Yes	15 (31.3)	9 (18.0)	$Chi^2 = 2.33$ $p = 0.13$
No	33 (68.8)	41 (82.0)	
Current medications, n (%)			
Yes	5 (10.4)	2 (4.0)	$Chi^2 = 1.52$ $p = 0.22$
No	43 (89.6)	43 (86.0)	
Experience with E-Mental Health, n (%)			
Yes, good	5 (10.4)	4 (8.0)	$Chi^2 = 0.17$ $p = 0.68$
Yes, bad	0 (0.0)	0 (0.0)	
No	43 (89.6)	46 (92.0)	

Table 3. Treatment Outcomes. Observed and Estimated Means for Primary and Secondary Outcome Measures and Within- and Between-Group effect-sizes.

	Pre-Treatment	Post-Treatment (Observed)		Post-Treatment (Estimated)		Follow-Up (Observed)		Post-Treatment Between-Group Comparisons (Group by Time)	Pre-Post Within-Group Effect Sizes (Estimated, ** for $p \leq 0.01$)	Between-Group Effect Sizes at Post (Est.)	
Measure	*n*	M (SD)	*n*	M (SD)	*n*	M (SE)	*n*	M (SD)	F and df	Cohen's *d* (95% CI)	Cohen's *d* (95% CI)
ADNM-20 Preoccupation											
CAU	50	13.12 (1.79)	35	11.41 (1.99)	50	11.70 (2.01)			$F_{1,96} = 0.03$	0.69 (0.47–0.91)	0.03 (−0.43–0.50)
Intervention	48	12.23 (2.22)	16	11.50 (2.15)	48	11.63 (2.27)	12	10.17 (2.37)		0.27 (0.09–0.45)	
ADNM-20 Failure to adapt											
CAU	50	9.85 (2.73)	35	8.68 (2.30)	50	8.66 (2.29)			$F_{1,96} = 3.13$	0.37 (0.18–0.57)	0.40 (−0.07–0.87)
Intervention	48	9.35 (2.12)	16	7.75 (2.25)	48	7.88 (2.09)	12	7.92 (2.07)		0.74 (0.52–0.93)	
ADNM-20 Accessory symptoms											
CAU	50	31.42 (5.70)	35	28.05 (4.82)	50	28.32 (5.41)			$F_{1,96} = 0.33$	0.55 (0.36–0.75)	0.51 (0.02–1.00)
Intervention	48	28.00 (6.37)	16	25.32 (6.64)	48	25.35 (6.38)	12	22.75 (5.85)		0.41 (0.18–0.63)	
BDI											
CAU	50	11.78 (3.87)	35	9.86 (4.44)	50	11.20 (4.78)			$F_{1,96} = 19.52$ **	0.13 (−0.06–0.31)	0.83 (0.41–1.25)
Intervention	48	10.83 (5.13)	16	9.76 (6.72)	48	10.23 (4.80)	12	4.44 (4.90)		0.72 (0.48–0.97)	
BSI-18											
CAU	50	12.52 (8.87)	35	11.41 (8.67)	50	10.80 (7.72)			$F_{1,96} = 0.49$	0.20 (0.02–0.39)	0.17 (−0.24–0.57)
Intervention	48	14.56 (9.18)	16	11.08 (6.22)	48	12.17 (8.72)	12	5.27 (5.46)		0.27 (0.14–0.39)	
SF-12_{PH}											
CAU	50	14.62 (3.34)	35	14.79 (3.29)	50	14.52 (3.15)			$F_{1,96} = 3.16$	−0.03 (−0.22–0.15)	0.36 (−0.04–0.76)
Intervention	48	14.60 (3.09)	16	15.20 (3.12)	48	15.60 (2.88)	12	18.00 (2.68)		0.33 (0.09-0.58)	
SF-12_{MH}											
CAU	50	15.96 (2.58)	35	15.68 (2.25)	50	15.96 (2.47)			$F_{1,96} = 13.52$ **	0.02 (−0.24–0.27)	0.74 (0.32–1.16)
Intervention	48	16.98 (2.62)	16	17.73 (2.40)	48	17.77 (2.40)	12	18.36 (2.01)		0.31 (0.07–0.55)	

For the primary outcome, the effect of the ADNM-20 was not qualified by significant Group × Time interactions for either the sum score ($F_{1,96} = 2.38$, p = ns), or for the subscales ($F_{1,96} = 0.03–3.13$, p = ns; see Table 3), meaning that the symptom severity did not decrease significantly in the intervention group compared to the control group. Between-group effect sizes based on estimated means, corrected for baseline differences, were small for the sum score ($d = 0.31$) and small to medium sized for the subscales ($d = 0.03–0.51$; see Table 3). Within-group comparisons based on estimated means in the treatment group showed large effect sizes for the sum score ($d = 1.04$) and small to medium effect sizes for the subscales ($d = 0.27–0.74$; see Table 3). Within-group effect sizes in the control group were medium-sized for the sum score ($d = 0.70$) and small to medium-sized as well for the subscales ($d = 0.37–0.69$; see Table 3).

As for secondary outcomes, the effect of the BDI showed significant Group × Time interactions (BDI: $F_{1,96} = 19.5$ $p < 0.01$). At post, between-group effect sizes based on estimated means were $d = 0.89$, meaning that for the intervention group, there was a large effect in terms of depressive symptom decrease compared to the control group. Within-group comparisons based on the estimated means in the treatment group showed large effect sizes (BDI: $d = 0.95$). In contrast, within-group effect sizes in the control group were negligible (BDI: $d = 0.20$). Treatment effects for the intervention group at three-month-follow-up were stable (pre–follow-up, $d = 0.95$) as no significant differences could be detected in comparison to the effects at post ($p > 0.30$).

For the SF-12 mental health subscale, there was a significant Group × Time interaction (SF-12_{MH}: $F_{1,96} = 13.52$, $p < 0.01$). At post, between-group effect sizes based on estimated means were $d = 0.74$, meaning that for the intervention group, there was a medium effect in terms of increased mental health-related quality of life compared to the control group at post. Within-group comparisons based on the estimated means in the treatment group showed small effect sized at post (SF-12_{MH_post}: $d = 0.31$) and significantly improved to medium effect size at follow-up (SF-12_{MH_fu}: $d = 0.68$, $p < 0.01$). In contrast, within-group effect sizes in the control group were negligible at post (SF-12_{MH}: $d = 0.02$). For the SF-12 physical health subscale, there were no significant Group × Time interactions detected (SF-12_{PH}: $F_{1,96} = 3.16$, $p = 0.08$).

3.4. Diagnostic Status Pre- and Post-Treatment

In total, 51 participants filled out the post-treatment questionnaire (Active, $n = 16$ (33%), CAU, $n = 35$ (70%)). According to the self-report at post-treatment, 15 out of 48 participants in the intervention group (31%) did not meet the criteria for AjD. In contrast, 14 participants in the control group (28%) could be considered remitted after four weeks.

3.5. Program Usage and Usability

The intensity in which the intervention was used shows a high degree of heterogeneity within the user group. The average time spent in the intervention (total) was 43 min (SD = 106.6), while the average duration of a session was 8 min (SD = 11). The average number of sessions (total) was 2.7 (SD = 5.2). The usability of the intervention was rated as above average by the users. The average SUS score was 73 (SD = 18), which translates to an adjective rating of "good" [51].

3.6. Predictors of Outcome

To investigate potential predictors of outcome, we used regression analyses, predicting 4-week primary and secondary outcomes, controlled for baseline scores. For these analyses, we only used data of participants that logged in at least once and completed the post-treatment questionnaires. None of the pre-treatment variables such as age, sex, marital status, occupational situation, education or psychotherapeutic treatment had any significant relation to the primary outcome (all $ps > 0.24$). At the same time, none of the indicators of program usage such as number of sessions or time spent in the intervention were significantly associated with the treatment outcomes for both groups of participants (all $ps > 0.27$).

4. Discussion

The present research aimed to develop a self-guided intervention for adjustment problems and to test its efficacy compared to a control group. Contrary to our hypothesis, there were no significant differences between the intervention group and the control group regarding the primary outcome measure ADNM-20 and its subscales. Both groups showed significantly lower AjD symptom burden from baseline to post-treatment. This result and the within-group effect size of d = 1.04 in the treatment group are in line with the results obtained with the original manual by Bachem and Maercker, what indicates its adequate online implementation [32,33]. The between-group effect size of d = 0.31 was not significant, whereas, the study was underpowered to detect small effects like this.

Although both groups showed similar improvements for the primary outcome, the intervention group showed a significant between-group effect on the reduction of depressive symptoms (d = 0.89). Effects within the intervention group could also be maintained over the three-month follow-up period. This is an encouraging result, which could not yet be shown in previous studies on internet interventions for AjD [22].

Likewise, there was a significant between-group effect regarding the improvement of mental health-related quality of life at post (d = 0.74). Within-group comparisons in the intervention group showed significant improvements over all three points of measurement, respectively (SF-12_{MH_post}: d = 0.31, SF-12_{MH_fu}: d = 0.68). For the physically related quality of life, there were no significant effects detected (SF-12_{PH}: d = 0.33, p = 0.08), which again could be related to the lack of power to detect small effect sizes in the present study.

The overall results are further consistent with those of the BADI self-guided approach to AjD treatment by Eimontas et al. [22]. It showed medium effect sizes regarding the AjD symptom reduction, starting from a comparable severity of symptom burden in the pre-treatment evaluation. In contrast to the present study, however, the control group showed no comparable improvements.

In a wider context, the results of the present study stand in accordance with previous research that supports the viability of self-guided approaches in different contexts [52,53]. We were able to show that highly scalable self-guided interventions have a positive effect on users. However, the effects are still small and many dropouts can be expected.

4.1. Limitations

Several limitations to this study need to be acknowledged. First, the sample consisted of self-selected participants. It can be assumed that already a positive opinion regarding internet interventions prevailed. This restricts generalizability, but on the flipside, also reflects a realistic health care scenario. Second, the study suffers from a high dropout rate of 48% (pre-post). Third, the results of the study are solely based on self-report measures, which however allows for scalability of the approach. Fourth, we had a relatively heterogeneous sample of participants regarding symptom burden. Fifth, unexpectedly, the organizational- and time-restrictions of the project did not allow the recruitment efforts to be extended in such a way as to achieve the number of participants required for the assumed effects. This calls for changes in future studies and restricts the generalizability of the current results, demanding their appropriately cautious interpretation. Lastly, from an ethical perspective, we deemed it important to not extend the delay for the waiting list further than needed in the potential period of onset of AjD as a transient disorder. However, this not only made a comparison between experimental and control group at three months impossible, but also clearly limits the informative value on account of the temporal stability of effect beyond this period.

4.2. Implications and Learnings

Even though it is an empirically common phenomenon, especially for self-guided interventions, the low adherence to the intervention, respectively high dropout of the participants, should not be overlooked. Several studies have already demonstrated meaningful relation to treatment outcome [22,54]. Thus, it is a positive sign, that significant effects have been found for ZIEL, despite the relatively small "adherence-dosage". However, a solution-oriented approach to the problem is mandatory and represents an important aspect of the further development of the intervention. We have to assume that we were not able to match the needs of users, e.g., in terms of technical or content-related aspects [55].

To improve adherence, we see different steps that could be implemented in the next iteration [56]. First, the integration of automated reminders should be able to increase engagement [57]. Complementary to this, the addition of automatic feedback on tasks and virtual rewards for favorable actions could be a valuable investment that we want to pursue. On a more general level, we see the need to improve the product-market-fit of the intervention in the broadest sense. To better be able to match user needs, we plan to focus and collaborate with specific target groups, based on classes of AjD-relevant life events like e.g., divorce. This would make it possible to generate greater personal relevance for the user on the one hand. On the other hand, we could target specific needs more directly and learn faster from focused user feedback. An example of such an approach in a guided format is the internet-based intervention for adaption problems after separation or divorce, called LIVIA, which showed significant improvements and moderate effect sizes for participants [58].

A positive and fruitful experience which we gained during the work on the present study, was with the closed loop between the development of both the content and the software. While there is currently a trend in our field towards outsourcing the technical implementation, it has proven very efficient for us to understand the content and IT as two sides of the same coin. Based on an agile strategy, one can make early decisive decisions for later developments. In other words, the hope is that initial investment in interdisciplinary teams will pay off several times over, in the lifecycle of fruitful projects. The approach becomes even more relevant in an academic context, with a multitude of parallel projects, changing financing situations and continuously changing teams.

In conclusion, the present study supports the current positive findings of efficient internet-based treatment of AjD. It expands the current state of knowledge with an extension of possible approaches to treatment and conceptual considerations regarding the process of realization. Given the potential reach and impact of a low threshold, high scalability intervention for AjD, sustainable research efforts are required.

Author Contributions: R.B. and A.M. developed the original intervention manual and its theoretical framework. C.M. developed the intervention platform and revised the content. A.M. and T.B. were involved in planning and supervised the work. C.M. wrote the manuscript with input from all authors.

Conflicts of Interest: The authors declare no conflict of interest.

Appendix A

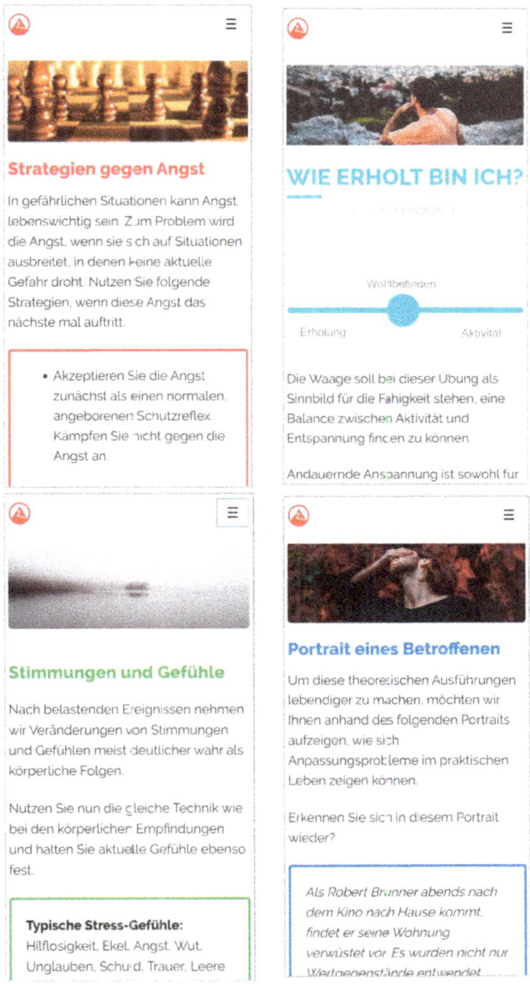

Figure A1. Illustrative Screenshots of the ZIEL Intervention.

References

1. Stoker, A. *Dracula*; Archibald Constable & Company: Dublin, OH, USA, 1897.
2. Casey, P.; Bailey, S. Adjustment disorders: The state of the art. *World Psychiatry* **2011**, *10*, 11–18. [CrossRef]
3. Keeley, J.W.; Reed, G.M.; Roberts, M.C.; Evans, S.C.; Robles, R.; Matsumoto, C.; Brewin, C.R.; Cloitre, M.; Perkonigg, A.; Rousseau, C.; et al. Disorders specifically associated with stress: A case-controlled field study for ICD-11 mental and behavioural disorders. *Int. J. Clin. Health Psychol.* **2016**, *16*, 109–127. [CrossRef] [PubMed]
4. Bachem, R.; Casey, P. Adjustment disorder: A diagnosis whose time has come. *J. Affect. Disord.* **2018**, *227*, 243–253. [CrossRef] [PubMed]
5. Evans, S.C.; Reed, G.M.; Roberts, M.C.; Esparza, P.; Watts, A.D.; Correia, J.M.; Ritchie, P.; May, M.; Saxena, S. Psychologists' perspectives on the diagnostic classification of mental disorders: Results from the WHO-IUPsyS Global Survey. *Int. J. Psychol.* **2013**, *48*, 177–193. [CrossRef] [PubMed]

6. Casey, P. *Adjustment Disorders: From Controversy to Clinical Practice*; Oxford University Press: Oxford, UK, 2018.
7. Strain, J.J.; Diefenbacher, A. The adjustment disorders: The conundrums of the diagnoses. *Compr. Psychiatry* **2008**, *49*, 121–130. [CrossRef] [PubMed]
8. World Health Organization. *The ICD-10 Classification of Mental and Behavioural Disorders: Clinical Descriptions and Diagnostic Guidelines*; World Health Organization: Geneva, Switzerland, 1992.
9. Association, A.P. *Diagnostic and Statistical Manual of Mental Disorders (DSM-5®)*; American Psychiatric Pub: Washington, DC, USA, 2013.
10. Casey, P.; Maracy, M.; Kelly, B.D.; Lehtinen, V.; Ayuso-Mateos, J.L.; Dalgard, O.S.; Dowrick, C. Can adjustment disorder and depressive episode be distinguished? Results from ODIN. *J. Affect. Disord.* **2006**, *92*, 291–297. [CrossRef] [PubMed]
11. Polyakova, I.; Knobler, H.Y.; Ambrumova, A.; Lerner, V. Characteristics of suicidal attempts in major depression versus adjustment reactions. *J. Affect. Disord.* **1998**, *47*, 159–167. [CrossRef]
12. O'Donnell, M.L.; Alkemade, N.; Creamer, M.; McFarlane, A.C.; Silove, D.; Bryant, R.A.; Felmingham, K.; Steel, Z.; Forbes, D. A longitudinal study of adjustment disorder after trauma exposure. *Am. J. Psychiatry* **2016**, *173*, 1231–1238. [CrossRef] [PubMed]
13. Runeson, B.S.; Beskow, J.; Waern, M. The suicidal process in suicides among young people. *Acta Psychiatr. Scand.* **1996**, *93*, 35–42. [CrossRef]
14. World Health Organization. *International Statistical Classification of Diseases and Related Health Problems*; World Health Organization: Geneva, Switzerland, 2018.
15. Carta, M.G.; Balestrieri, M.; Murru, A.; Hardoy, M.C. Adjustment Disorder: Epidemiology, diagnosis and treatment. *Clin. Pract. Epidemiol. Ment. Health* **2009**, *5*, 15. [CrossRef]
16. Strain, J.J.; Smith, G.C.; Hammer, J.S.; McKenzie, D.P.; Blumenfield, M.; Muskin, P.; Newstadt, G.; Wallack, J.; Wilner, A.; Schleifer, S.S. Adjustment disorder: A multisite study of its utilization and interventions in the consultation-liaison psychiatry setting. *Gen. Hosp. Psychiatry* **1998**, *20*, 139–149. [CrossRef]
17. Dalgaard, L.; Eskildsen, A.; Carstensen, O.; Willert, M.V.; Andersen, J.H.; Glasscock, D.J. Changes in self-reported sleep and cognitive failures: A randomized controlled trial of a stress management intervention. *Scand. J. Work Environ. Health* **2014**, *40*, 569–581. [CrossRef] [PubMed]
18. Cvetek, R. EMDR treatment of distressful experiences that fail to meet the criteria for PTSD. *J. EMDR Pract. Res.* **2008**, *2*, 2. [CrossRef]
19. Altenhöfer, A.; Schulz, W.; Schwab, R.; Eckert, J. Psychotherapie von Anpassungsstörungen. *Psychotherapeut* **2007**, *52*, 24–34. [CrossRef]
20. Gabbard, G.O. *Gabbard's Treatments of Psychiatric Disorders*; American Psychiatric Pub: Washington, DC, USA, 2007.
21. Baños, R.M.; Guillen, V.; Quero, S.; Garcia-Palacios, A.; Alcaniz, M.; Botella, C. A virtual reality system for the treatment of stress-related disorders: A preliminary analysis of efficacy compared to a standard cognitive behavioral program. *Int. J. Hum. Comput. Stud.* **2011**, *69*, 602–613. [CrossRef]
22. Eimontas, J.; Rimsaite, Z.; Gegieckaite, G.; Zelviene, P.; Kazlauskas, E. Internet-based self-help intervention for ICD-11 adjustment disorder: Preliminary findings. *Psychiatr. Q.* **2018**, *89*, 451–460. [CrossRef] [PubMed]
23. Rachyla, I.; Quero Castellano, S.; Pérez Ara, M.Á.; Molés Amposta, M.; Campos, D.; Mira Pastor, A. *Web-Based, Self-Help Intervention for Adjustment Disorders: Acceptance and Usability*; Interactive Media Institute (IMI): San Diego, CA, USA, 2017.
24. Lindsäter, E.; Axelsson, E.; Salomonsson, S.; Santoft, F.; Ejeby, K.; Ljótsson, B.; Akerstedt, T.; Lekander, M.; Hedman-Lagerlöf, E. Internet-Based Cognitive Behavioral Therapy for Chronic Stress: A Randomized Controlled Trial. *Psychother. Psychosom.* **2018**, *87*, 296–305. [CrossRef] [PubMed]
25. Berger, T. *Internetbasierte Interventionen bei Psychischen Störungen*; Hogrefe Verlag: Göttingen, Germany, 2015.
26. Maercker, A.; Bachem, R.C.; Lorenz, L.; Moser, C.T.; Berger, T. Adjustment disorders are uniquely suited for ehealth interventions: Concept and case study. *JMIR Ment. Health* **2015**, *2*, e15. [CrossRef]
27. Gega, L.; Marks, I.; Mataix-Cols, D. Computer-aided CBT self-help for anxiety and depressive disorders: Experience of a London clinic and future directions. *J. Clin. Psychol.* **2004**, *60*, 147–157. [CrossRef]
28. Petersen, K.; Wohlin, C. The effect of moving from a plan-driven to an incremental software development approach with agile practices. *Empir. Softw. Eng.* **2010**, *15*, 654–693. [CrossRef]
29. Christensen, H.; Griffiths, K. The Internet and mental health literacy. *Aust. N. Z. J. Psychiatry* **2000**, *34*, 975–979. [CrossRef] [PubMed]

30. Christensen, H.; Petrie, K. Information technology as the key to accelerating advances in mental health care. *Aust. N. Z. J. Psychiatry* **2013**, *47*, 114–116. [CrossRef] [PubMed]
31. ClinicalTrials.gov. Identifier NCT03379155. Available online: https://clinicaltrials (accessed on 28 August 2019).
32. SealedEnvelope.com. Available online: www.sealedenvelope (accessed on 28 August 2019).
33. Bootstrap. Open Source Toolkit for Developing with HTML, CSS, and JS. 2019. Available online: www.getbootstrap (accessed on 28 August 2019).
34. Bachem, R.; Maercker, A. *Ist das Noch Mein Zuhause*; Mobiliar Versicherung: Bern, Switzerland, 2013.
35. Bachem, R.; Maercker, A. Self-help interventions for adjustment disorder problems: A randomized waiting-list controlled study in a sample of burglary victims. *Cogn. Behav. Ther.* **2016**, *45*, 397–413. [CrossRef] [PubMed]
36. Glaesmer, H.; Romppel, M.; Brähler, E.; Hinz, A.; Maercker, A. Adjustment disorder as proposed for ICD-11: Dimensionality and symptom differentiation. *Psychiatry Res.* **2015**, *229*, 940–948. [CrossRef] [PubMed]
37. Einsle, F.; Köllner, V.; Dannemann, S.; Maercker, A. Development and validation of a self-report for the assessment of adjustment disorders. *Psychol. Health Med.* **2010**, *15*, 584–595. [CrossRef] [PubMed]
38. Lorenz, L.; Bachem, R.C.; Maercker, A. The adjustment disorder–new module 20 as a screening instrument: Cluster analysis and cut-off values. *Int. J. Occup. Environ. Med. (IJOEM)* **2016**, *7*, 215–220. [CrossRef] [PubMed]
39. Spitzer, C.; Hammer, S.; Löwe, B.; Grabe, H.J.; Barnow, S.; Rose, M.; Wingenfeld, K.; Freyberger, H.J.; Franke, G.H. The short version of the Brief Symptom Inventory (BSI-18): Preliminary psychometric properties of the German translation. *Fortschr. Neurol. Psychiatr.* **2011**, *79*, 517–523. [CrossRef] [PubMed]
40. Beck, A.T.; Ward, C.H.; Mendelson, M.; Mock, J.; Erbaugh, J. An inventory for measuring depression. *Arch. Gen. Psychiatry* **1961**, *4*, 561–571. [CrossRef]
41. Beck, A.T.; Steer, R.A.; Carbin, M.G. Psychometric properties of the Beck Depression Inventory: Twenty-five years of evaluation. *Clin. Psychol. Rev.* **1988**, *8*, 77–100. [CrossRef]
42. Ware, J.E.; Kosinski, M.; Keller, S.D. A 12-Item Short-Form Health Survey: Construction of Scales and Preliminary Tests of Reliability and Validity. *Med Care* **1996**, *34*, 220–233. [CrossRef]
43. Gandek, B.; Ware, J.E.; Aaronson, N.K.; Apolone, G.; Bjorner, J.B.; Brazier, J.E.; Bullinger, M.; Kaasa, S.; Leplege, A.; Prieto, L.; et al. Cross-validation of item selection and scoring for the SF-12 Health Survey in nine countries: Results from the IQOLA Project. *J. Clin. Epidemiol.* **1998**, *51*, 1171–1178. [CrossRef]
44. Devilly, G.J.; Borkovec, T.D. Psychometric properties of the credibility/expectancy questionnaire. *J. Behav. Ther. Exp. Psychiatry* **2000**, *31*, 73–86. [CrossRef]
45. Jordan, P.W.; Thomas, B.; McClelland, I.L.; Weerdmeester, B. *Usability Evaluation in Industry*; CRC Press: Boca Raton, FL, USA, 1996.
46. Brooke, J. SUS-A quick and dirty usability scale. *Usability Eval. Ind.* **1996**, *189*, 4–7.
47. Faul, F.; Erdfelder, E.; Buchner, A.; Lang, A.G. Statistical power analyses using G* Power 3.1: Tests for correlation and regression analyses. *Behav. Res. Methods* **2009**, *41*, 1149–1160. [CrossRef]
48. Gueorguieva, R.; Krystal, J.H. Move over anova: Progress in analyzing repeated-measures data andits reflection in papers published in the archives of general psychiatry. *Arch. Gen. Psychiatry* **2004**, *61*, 310–317. [CrossRef] [PubMed]
49. Team, R.C. *R: A Language and Environment for Statistical Computing*; R Foundation for Statistical Computing: Vienna, Austria, 2016.
50. Bates, D.; Mächler, M.; Bolker, B.; Walker, S. Fitting linear mixed-effects models using lme4. *arXiv* **2014**, arXiv:1406.5823.
51. Bangor, A.; Kortum, P.; Miller, J. Determining what individual SUS scores mean: Adding an adjective rating scale. *J. Usability Stud.* **2009**, *4*, 114–123.
52. Karyotaki, E.; Riper, H.; Twisk, J.; Hoogendoorn, A.; Kleiboer, A.; Mira, A.; Mackinnon, A.; Meyer, B.; Botella, C.; Littlewood, E.; et al. Efficacy of self-guided internet-based cognitive behavioral therapy in the treatment of depressive symptoms: A meta-analysis of individual participant data. *JAMA Psychiatry* **2017**, *74*, 351–359. [CrossRef]
53. Berger, T.; Hämmerli, K.; Gubser, N.; Andersson, G.; Caspar, F. Internet-based treatment of depression: A randomized controlled trial comparing guided with unguided self-help. *Cogn. Behav. Ther.* **2011**, *40*, 251–266. [CrossRef]

54. Rachyla, I.; Pérez-Ara, M.; Molés, M.; Campos, D.; Mira, A.; Botella, C.; Quero, S. An internet-based intervention for adjustment disorder (TAO): Study protocol for a randomized controlled trial. *BMC Psychiatry* **2018**, *18*, 161. [CrossRef]
55. Christensen, H.; Griffiths, K.M.; Farrer, L. Adherence in internet interventions for anxiety and depression: Systematic review. *J. Med. Internet Res.* **2009**, *11*, e13. [CrossRef] [PubMed]
56. Baumel, A.; Birnbaum, M.L.; Sucala, M. A systematic review and taxonomy of published quality criteria related to the evaluation of user-facing eHealth programs. *J. Med. Syst.* **2017**, *41*, 128. [CrossRef] [PubMed]
57. Fogg, B.J. A behavior model for persuasive design. In Proceedings of the 4th international Conference on Persuasive Technology, Claremont, CA, USA, 26–29 April 2009; p. 40.
58. Brodbeck, J.; Berger, T.; Biesold, N.; Rockstroh, F.; Znoj, H.J. Evaluation of a guided internet-based self-help intervention for older adults after spousal bereavement or separation/divorce: A randomised controlled trial. *J. Affect. Disord.* **2019**, *252*, 440–449. [CrossRef] [PubMed]

Journal of
Clinical Medicine

MDPI

Article

Analysis of Usage Data from a Self-Guided App-Based Virtual Reality Cognitive Behavior Therapy for Acrophobia: A Randomized Controlled Trial

Tara Donker [1,2,3,*], Chris van Klaveren [4], Ilja Cornelisz [4], Robin N. Kok [5,6] and Jean-Louis van Gelder [7,8]

1 Department of Clinical, Neuro and Developmental Psychology, Section Clinical Psychology, Vrije Universiteit Amsterdam, Van der Boechorststraat 1, 1081 BT Amsterdam, The Netherlands
2 Amsterdam Public Health Research Institute Amsterdam, Van der Boechorststraat 7, 1081 BT Amsterdam, The Netherlands
3 Department of Psychology, Laboratory of Biological and Personality Psychology, Albert Ludwigs-University of Freiburg, Peter-Kaplan Meierstrasse 8, 79104 Freiburg im Breisgau, Germany
4 Department of Education Sciences, Section Methods and Statistics and Amsterdam Center for Learning Analytics, Vrije Universiteit Amsterdam, Van der Boechorststraat 1, 1081 BT Amsterdam, The Netherlands; c.p.b.j.van.klaveren@vu.nl (C.v.K.); i.cornelisz@vu.nl (I.C.)
5 Department of Psychology, University of Southern Denmark, Campusvej 55, 5230 Odense, Denmark; rkok@health.sdu.dk
6 Centre for Innovative Medical Technology, Odense University Hospital, Indgang 101, 5000 Odense, Denmark
7 Institute of Education and Child Studies, Leiden University, Pieter de la Court building, 4th floor, Wassenaarseweg 52, 2333 AK Leiden, The Netherlands; jlvangelder@gmail.com
8 Max Planck Institute for the Study of Crime, Security and Law, Department of Criminology, Günterstalstraße 73, 79100 Freiburg, Germany
* Correspondence: t.donker@vu.nl; Tel.: +31-20-5988959; Fax: +31-20-5988758

Received: 10 April 2020; Accepted: 22 May 2020; Published: 26 May 2020

Abstract: This study examined user engagement with ZeroPhobia, a self-guided app-based virtual reality (VR) Cognitive Behavior Therapy for acrophobia symptoms using cardboard VR viewers. Dutch acrophobic adults (n = 96) completed assessments at baseline and immediately following treatment. Primary outcome measures were the Acrophobia Questionnaire (AQ) and the Igroup Presence Questionnaire (IPQ). Usage data consisted of number of VR sessions practiced, practice time, and fear ratings directly after practicing. Results show that of the 66 participants who played at least one level, the majority continued to finish all levels, spending on average 24.4 min in VR. Self-reported fear consistently decreased between the start and finish of levels. Post-test AQ scores depended quadratically on time spent in VR. Higher pre-test AQ scores were significantly associated with subjective anxiety after the first level and a reduction of post-test AQ scores, but not with number of sessions, suggesting it might be more beneficial to play one level for a longer time period instead of practicing many VR levels. Results also show an optimum exposure level at which increasing practice time does not result in increased benefit. Self-guided VR acrophobia treatment is effective and leads to consistent reductions in self-reported anxiety both between levels and after treatment. Most participants progressed effectively to the highest self-exposure level, despite the absence of a therapist.

Keywords: acrophobia; cognitive behaviour therapy; mobile app; virtual reality; usage data

1. Introduction

Given the global challenge of access to evidence-based psychological treatment for common mental health disorders, there is an evident need for affordable and scalable self-help interventions [1]. Reasons for limited access include a lack of mental health professionals and high treatment costs [2]. Digital interventions may offer a solution. Several meta-analyses of randomized controlled trials (RCTs) have demonstrated effectiveness for digital interventions, mostly online, for treating common mental disorders such as anxiety disorders [3–5]. Innovations in this field comprise virtual reality (VR) and mobile applications (apps) [2]. There is empirical evidence that such interventions can be similar in effectiveness compared to face-to-face treatment [1,6–10]. For example, Morina et al. [9] demonstrated in their meta-analysis that results of behavioral assessment at post-treatment and at follow-up revealed no significant differences between VRET and exposure in vivo. Furthermore, in our study [1] we showed that results of an VR-CBT-based app were comparable to results found in studies investigating the effectiveness of traditional CBT. However, less is known about how user adherence and engagement relates to effectiveness of these interventions, especially with regard to VR and mobile app-based interventions. One exception is the study of Hong et al. [11] in which the effectiveness and usage of a mobile-based self-training VR program for acrophobia was investigated. Interestingly, heart rate (HR) and gaze down percentage were also included in this study. Using a pre-post study design with two arms (high and low acrophobic symptoms), Hong et al. demonstrated that participants with higher acrophobia symptoms derived more benefit from the VR program compared to those with lower acrophobia symptoms. Furthermore, they found a negative correlation with gaze-down percentage in the high acrophobia symptom group compared to the low acrophobia symptom group. In this study, subjects attended a VR-center and had contact with research staff. Treatment efficiency and effectiveness could be enhanced by a better understanding of how intervention usage affects outcome [12–14]. For example, treatment efficiency can be improved through the identification of redundant elements that do not contribute to symptom reduction. Treatment effectiveness can be increased by identifying where participants drop-out and improving that element to reduce drop-out. Exploring usage data of fully self-guided interventions is of particular importance due to the lack of human oversight and the resulting inability to adjust the course of such interventions [12]. An analysis of usage data can be beneficial in optimizing the uptake and continued use of these self-guided interventions.

Recent studies examining usage data of digital interventions have demonstrated that highly active users completing more modules predict better outcomes for eating disorders, smoking cessation and depression [15–19]. Previous studies also demonstrated that higher activity during the first week of treatment is a predictor of better adherence for web-based interventions [20,21]. Moreover, more concise and shorter interventions achieve better usage rates compared to extensive interventions [22]. However, in a recent review, Donkin et al. [15] concluded that several potential usage metrics (number of log-ins, time spent online) were inconsistently associated with outcomes for online interventions for psychological disorders. Only the relation between proportion of completed modules and outcome emerged as a consistent association [15,16]. Previous research into VR treatment indicated that presence plays an important role in the effectiveness of a program [23]). For example, in our study reporting the main results of this trial we found that a larger reduction in acrophobia symptoms was associated when the feeling of being present in the virtual environment was higher [1].

The efficacy of VR interventions for acrophobia has been well-documented (for an overview, see [24]. However, with few exceptions (e.g., [25]) usage data of virtual reality (mobile app) interventions for common mental disorders has remained largely unexplored. For self-guided VR interventions, participant retention is important as there is no therapist oversight into the process. The aim of the present study was to examine usage of, and engagement, with, ZeroPhobia, a fully self-guided app-based virtual reality Cognitive Behavior Therapy (VR-CBT) for acrophobia, using mobile phones and a low-cost (cardboard) virtual reality viewer, and to determine user metrics contributing to effectiveness. The most important element of CBT for anxiety disorders is exposure, in which the participant is repeatedly confronted with the feared object or situation, thus learning that the expected disaster is not happening. This, in turn, leads to decreases in anxiety symptoms [26]. We specified the following exploratory hypotheses: (1) higher VR activity (number of completed VR sessions, practice time in VR) is associated with reduced post-test acrophobia symptoms; (2) higher presence scores on the IPQ are correlated with stronger decreases in anxiety ratings directly after practicing with exposure in the VR environment; (3) higher acrophobia symptoms at pre-test correlate positively with VR anxiety ratings and VR activity, and negatively with a reduction in acrophobia symptoms at post-test; and (4) post-session anxiety levels consistently decrease compared to pre-session anxiety levels after repeated practice in the VR environment.

2. Materials and Methods

2.1. Study Design and Procedure

In the current study, we carried out a secondary analysis of a previously published outcome study [1]. Details of the materials and methods are described elsewhere and will therefore not be dealt with in detail here [1,27]. In short, in this single-blind RCT, participants were recruited from the Dutch general population through websites, magazines and local media. Ethical approval was received from the Medical Ethics Committee of the VU University Medical Center (registration number 2016-563, Trial registration: NTR6442) [1]. Participants were randomized into two groups: intervention or waitlist. The research team was blind to treatment allocation. All materials were completed online without researcher intervention. Trial Registration: Nederlands Trial Register http://www.trialregister.nl identifier: NTR6442 (prospectively registered).

2.2. Participants

Participants (18–65 years) who provided written informed consent by email or mail, who scored at least 45.45 on the Acrophobia Questionnaire (AQ)-Anxiety [28,29], had access to an Android smartphone (Android v.5.1 Lollipop or higher, 4.7–5.5 inch screen and gyroscope) were included in the study. Participants with insufficient Dutch language skills, or participants receiving current phobia treatment or psychotropic medication < 3 months were excluded from the study, as well as participants having severe depression (Patient Health Questionnaire [PHQ-9], [30]; total score > 19) or suicidality (Web Screening Questionnaire; WSQ, score ≥ 3; [31]). Enrollment commenced 24 March and ceased 28 September 2017.

2.3. Intervention: ZeroPhobia

ZeroPhobia-Acrophobia consists of six animated and engaging modules using 2D animations which provide background information and explain key concepts (e.g., the fear curve). The annimations are accompanied by an explanatory voice-over and an animated virtual therapist (modelled after the first author) about the nature and origins of the phobia, how to deal with it, setting goals, exercises, getting through difficult moments, cognitive behavioral therapy to deal with negative thoughts and practicing with challenging situations. The modules take between 5 and 40 min to complete. Exposure, the core of the treatment, is realized through gamified mobile VR and four 360° videos covering the entire acrophobia exposure spectrum. Participants started using the VR and the 360° videos from Module 3 onwards and navigated through the virtual environment using gaze control. Gaze control is a method for the hands-free selection of objects and the activation of functions within a virtual environment. By looking at an object or button in the center of the field of view for a specified period of time, e.g., 2 s, the object or button is selected or activated. In ZeroPhobia, large arrows served as interactive buttons used for navigating the virtual environment. By gazing at an arrow, a user moved to the location of the arrow. Similarly, items that needed to be collected, as part of the assignments in the various levels, could be selected by looking at them. The cardboard viewer could be strapped to the head. The VR involved a gamified virtual theater. In the game participants had to complete a series of increasingly challenging tasks (e.g., changing a light bulb on a small ladder, connecting speakers at the edge of the stage, going up a high ladder to repair a small damaged platform, fixing a spotlight on the highest balcony, saving a cat while being on a gangway high above the stage). In each level, participants had to look at assets located on the theatre floor that needed to be collected, hence encouraging them to look down and face their fears [27]. For more details on the VR environments used, see [1,27].

Because any VR setup that generates frame rates below 90 frames per seconds is likely to induce disorientation, nausea and other negative user effects, the frame rate was increased to an optimal level to minimize the risk of cybersickness. Furthermore, there were no quickly moving objects and it was not possible for the user to move quickly through the VR environment. Battery drainage was reduced by keeping the VR levels at an optimum duration meaning that playing a VR level did not exceed 10 min, although participants were at liberty to practice in VR as long as they felt like they needed. Battery drainage was further for small degree lessened indirectly by removing the back cover off the phone, which reduced overheating. The app provides safety instructions to participants before entering the VR environment. For example, participants were instructed to remove all sharp objects in their environment prior to commencing with VR-exposure, to avoid possible injuries. Also, they were instructed to start practicing in VR while seated. Only once anxiety decreased, participants were encouraged to practice standing up. They were also instructed to take off their VR viewer immediately if they felt they might fall.

For the current usage analyses, only information from the interactive VR environment was used, not the 360° videos. This is because the majority of participants were unable to view the 360° videos due to technical limitations of their smartphone (they encountered a black screen). They could, however, view the 360° videos on YouTube. The trial was delivered over a 3-week period during which participants were at liberty to practice with ZeroPhobia as often and as long as they wanted [1]. Weekly standardized motivational e-mails with reminders to start or continue with ZeroPhobia were sent to participants during the intervention period. For details, see [27] and for ZeroPhobia screenshots Figure S1. The VR environment was created with the Unity game engine (version 2017.3.0f3; Unity Technologies, San Francisco, CA, USA).

2.4. Outcomes

All questionnaires were completed online. Measures were taken at baseline (pre-test), immediately after the intervention (posttest), and 3 months after the intervention (follow-up). Participant characteristics measures were collected at baseline, while symptom measures were administered at each time point. All assessments were programmed with Survalyzer software [32]. See [27] for details on outcome measures. The primary outcome was the 20-item Acrophobia Questionnaire (AQ) [28]. The AQ is a widely-used validated instrument [29]. The anxiety subscale is measured using a 7-point Likert scale (0 = not anxious to 6 = extremely anxious). Total score ranges is 0–120. The avoidance subscale uses a 3-point Likert scale ("I would not avoid it" to "I would not do it under any circumstances"). Secondary outcomes included in this study were the Igroup Presence Questionnaire (IPQ); [33] to assess presence in VR, and usage. Because the IPQ is widely used in VR research and to be able to compare results on presence with previous studies, we chose the IPQ instead of other measures targeting presence. Usage data consisted of practice time in VR (for each level [time between entering and exiting the VR level] and in total [the sum of all practice time in VR per patient in minutes]), number of sessions (were one session is defined as repeatedly practicing with the same level) and anxiety ratings directly after practicing a session in the VR environment. As described in [27], participants were encouraged to progress to a more difficult level as soon as self-reported fear dropped below 4 on a 10-point scale. For self-reported fear between 4–7, participants were advised to try the same level again, and for self-reported fear levels 8–10 they were strongly advised to keep practicing the current level. Participants could not continue to the next level without self-reporting fear under 4.

2.5. Usage Data Retrieval

Usage data was retrieved from the ZeroPhobia app to a server which then stored the data on a database, on a secure (SSL) website. All communication between the app and the database was encrypted by means of a certificate. To prevent others (non-participants) from contaminating the database with data, adding new data was only possible by sending the correct key from one of the participants in the study. The data was pseudo-anonymized, meaning that data was anonymized but linked with the trial identifier consisting of four numbers. Examples of database reads are time spent in a VR level, time stamps (start and end time of a participant in the VR environment) that enabled us to exactly determine duration of practice time for each VR level, and experienced anxiety levels after each VR level played.

2.6. Statistical Analyses

Demographic and clinical characteristics are presented in terms of means and SDs. Usage data are presented in terms of means, SDs, and minimum and maximum observations for two groups: (1) all participants and (2) participants who have at least experienced one VR session. The primary outcome (AQ) was replicated using the same imputation methods and covariates as performed in Donker et al. [1], with the exception that the model was not estimated with CLS but instead with Maximum Likelihood Estimation. This estimation method is convenient as it allows parameterization of the treatment effect such that associations with the usage covariates can be directly estimated. Two-sided p-value < 0.05 indicated statistical significance. STATA version 14.2 (StataCorp LP., Texas, TX, USA) were used for the analyses. A data monitoring committee was not required by the Ethics Committee because of the expected low safety risk of the participants.

3. Results

3.1. Sample, Baseline Characteristics and Cybersickness

Details of the participant flow and drop-out are described elsewhere [1,27]. In short, of 663 individuals who signed up for participation, 291 were ineligible (e.g., due to phone ineligibility) and therefore excluded from participation. In total, 193 participants filled in the baseline assessment and were randomly assigned to the VR-CBT app condition (n = 96) or to the wait-list control condition. The pre-treatment attrition rate was 23% in the app condition because of illness (1 [1%]) or an incompatible smartphone (21 [22%]) [1]. Of the total sample (N = 96), the mean age was 41 years (SD = 13.73) and 66 (68.75%) of them were female. Most participants completed postsecondary education (n = 84; 87.5%). The mean AQ baseline score was 85.16 (SD: 18.42). Of the 96 randomized participants, 21 (23%) could not download ZeroPhobia on their smartphone because the smartphones were lacking a gyroscope (required for experiencing VR) and one (1%) did not start ZeroPhobia because of illness, leaving the sample with n = 74 participants.

3.2. General VR Usage Data

Of the 74 participants, 66 participants (68.8%) experienced at least one VR session. Usage data for these 66 participants are shown in Table 1, where the total VR duration time of active users is 24.4 min, with a minimum of 0.6 min (36 s) and a maximum of 71.05 min. On average, active participants practiced with around nine VR sessions. As can be seen, the anxiety ratings of participants are substantially different for practicing with level 1 compared to the highest level they attained (for most participants, this was level 5). The anxiety rating after playing a more difficult level, was on average lower than the anxiety rating after playing level one for the first time. When the anxiety ratings after playing a certain level for the first time were compared with anxiety ratings after playing a certain level for the last time (e.g., the anxiety rating after having played level 4 for the last time as compared to playing level 4 for the first time), we noted that anxiety was reduced by around 1.3 points on average (range: 1–10).

Table 1. Overall descriptive Statistics of Usage Data for Users who Experienced at least one VR session.

Variable	N	Mean	SD	Min	Max
Total					
Duration (total VR time in minutes)	66	24.384	16.127	0.600	71.050
Anxiety rating after playing level 1 [1]	66	3.545	2.288	1.000	10.000
Anxiety rating of highest attained level [2]	66	3.227	1.830	1.000	9.000
Anxiety rating after playing level first time [3]	66	4.576	2.308	1.000	10.000
Anxiety rating after playing level last time [4]	66	3.227	1.830	1.000	9.000
Number of VR sessions	66	9.167	5.365	2.000	25.000
Women					
Duration (total VR time in minutes) [1]	47	23.516	15.744	0.600	58.967
Anxiety rating after playing level 1 [2]	47	3.894	2.343	1.000	10.000
Anxiety rating of highest attained level [3]	47	3.149	1.818	1.000	9.000
Anxiety rating after playing level first time [4]	47	4.596	2.242	1.000	10.000
Anxiety rating after playing level last time [5]	47	3.149	1.818	1.000	9.000
Number of VR sessions	47	9.085	5.344	2.000	24.000
Men					
Duration (total VR time in minutes)	19	26.532	17.289	3.517	71.050
Anxiety rating after playing level 1 [2]	19	2.684	1.945	1.000	7.000
Anxiety rating of highest attained level [3]	19	3.421	1.895	1.000	9.000
Anxiety rating after playing level first time [4]	19	4.526	2.525	2.000	10.000
Anxiety rating after playing level last time [5]	19	3.421	1.895	1.000	9.000
Number of VR sessions	19	9.368	5.560	3.000	25.000

[1] Grubbs test was conducted to test for outliers and confirmed the apparent absence of outliers. Please see Figure S2 for details on the variation in practicing duration. [2] anxiety rating after playing level 1 (the easiest level: changing a light bulb on a small ladder) for the first time. [3] anxiety rating after playing the highest level (for that person) for the last time, which is level 5 for most participants (range: 1–10). [4] anxiety rating after playing a level for the first time [5] anxiety rating after playing a level for the last time (range: 1–10).

A paired t-test indicated that this difference was statistically significant (t (280) = 12.28, $p < 0.0001$) (see Table 2).

Table 2. Level-specific Statistics of Usage Data for Users who Experienced at least one VR session.

Variable	N	Mean	SD	Min	Max
LEVEL 1					
Time spent in level (minutes) [1]	65	2.289	2.109	0.317	11.483
Initial anxiety [2]	65	3.554	2.305	1	10
Final anxiety [3]	65	2.092	0.861	1	5
Number of sessions in level [4]	65	2.046	1.556	1	8
LEVEL2					
Time spent in level (minutes)	62	5.322	5.334	0.283	36.350
Initial anxiety	62	4.129	2.229	1	10
Final anxiety	62	2.645	1.527	1	10
Number of sessions in level	62	2.177	1.337	1	6
LEVEL 3					
Time spent in level (minutes)	57	7.768	5.222	0.967	23.367
Initial anxiety	57	5.070	2.638	1	10
Final anxiety	57	2.877	1.489	1	9
Number of sessions in level	57	2.281	1.278	1	7
LEVEL 4					
Time spent in level (minutes)	50	6.742	5.639	1.100	29.517
Initial anxiety	50	4.700	2.517	1	10
Final anxiety	50	2.940	1.096	1	7
Number of sessions in level	50	2.260	1.724	1	11

Table 2. *Cont.*

Variable	N	Mean	SD	Min	Max
LEVEL 5					
Time spent in level (minutes)	47	7.463	4.678	1.5	19.883
Initial anxiety	47	4.213	2.010	1	9
Final anxiety	47	2.872	1.035	1	7
Number of sessions in level	47	2.000	1.351	1	8
TOTAL					
Time spent in level (minutes)	281	5.727	5.114	0.233	36.350
Initial anxiety	281	4.302	2.397	1	10
Final anxiety	281	2.655	1.270	1	10
Number of sessions in level	281	2.153	1.450	1	11

[1] Total time spent in this level, in minutes. [2] Self-reported anxiety after playing this level for the first time (range: 1–10).[3] Self-reported anxiety after playing this level for the last time (range: 1–10).[4] Number of sessions spent in this level.

3.3. Level-Specific Usage Data

As can be seen in the level-specific usage results in Table 2, the self-reported anxiety of users was, on average, relatively low (M = 4.302, SD = 2.397) when finishing levels for the first time (initial anxiety). The final anxiety numbers show that on average, users exited a level with a self-reported anxiety level of 2.665 (SD = 1.270). This shows that most users complied well with the advice to 'level up' after self-reported anxiety had dropped below 3, however some users chose to replay a level up to 11 times (level 4).

3.4. Replication of Main Results

An intent-to-treat analysis showed a significant reduction of acrophobia symptoms at post-test at 3 months for ZeroPhobia compared with the controls ($b = -26.73$ [95%CI, −32.12 to −21.34]; $p < 0.001$; $d = 1.14$ [95%CI, 0.84 to 1.44]). Using the ML-estimation procedure, similar results for ZeroPhobia effectiveness were found compared to original study (b(SE) = −26.7 (2.73), noting a slight difference in standard error due to using a ML-estimation rather than an ordinary least squares approach as in [1].

3.5. Hypothesis 1: More VR Activity Is Associated With Lower Post-Test AQ Scores

To test the hypothesis that more VR activity is associated with a greater reduction in AQ scores at post-test, we modelled the post-test scores of the AQ with the pre-test scores on the AQ, the number of sessions played and a linear and quadratic parameter of practice time in minutes. The results show that practice time and the number of sessions result in lower post-test AQ scores, although number of sessions is not statistically significant. Post-test AQ scores depends quadratically on time spent practicing (Practice Time: b(SE) = −1.07(0.391); $p < 0.05$; PT^2: b(SE) = 0.018(0.005); $p < 0.05$). The association with number of sessions was not statistically significant. To test for robustness, this analysis was performed with and without baseline covariates in the model, but results did not change significantly. With respect to the estimated association between the number of sessions and Post-test AQ scores, we note that the inclusion of background characteristics does not change the estimated coefficient, but it does make the association insignificant. The insignificant result may be the result of lack of statistical power.

In Figure 1 the association between decrease in AQ scores and practice time and number of sessions is represented graphically, where darker areas denote a greater reduction in AQ scores at post-test. These results suggest the existence of a 'sweet spot', an optimum level of exposure at which increasing practice time does not result in an increased benefit and that it does not significantly depend on the number of sessions. The optimum level of practice time in the VR environment was found to be 25.5 min.

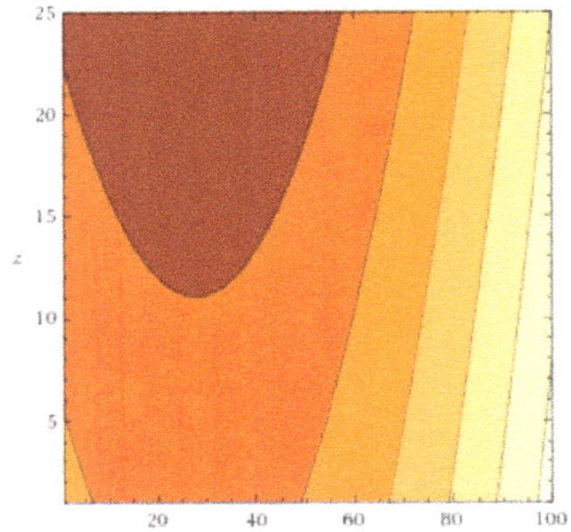

Figure 1. Practice Time (x-axis) vs. Number of Sessions (z-axis). Figure 1 visualizes the estimated function $AQ\_Total\_Post = -1.02x + 0.02x^2 - 1.17z - 12.85$ and plots a contour plot for $x = 1$ *to* 100 and $z = 1$ *to* 25. It thus represents a contour plot in which the outcome differences for the observed combinations of practice time (x-axis) and number of sessions (z-axis). The darker the color, the larger the outcome difference.

3.6. Hypothesis 2: A Higher Level of Presence Is Associated with Greater Decrease in Post-Session Anxiety

To test this hypothesis, we tested the association between the IPQ scores post-test and the treatment effect while controlling for baseline covariates. We also controlled for practice time, and pre-test AQ scores, as this would be associated with treatment effect. Because not all participants filled in the IPQ at post-test (12/66 missing, 21.2%), this variable was also modeled.

The results showed that those who filled out the IPQ, a higher level of presence was associated with a larger reduction of AQ scores post-test b(SE) = −0.914 (0.225), $p < 0.001$, confirming our hypothesis. The addition of the IPQ variable to the model did not change the parameter for the AQ pre-test scores, indicating that presence is not associated with pre-test AQ scores. The practice time coefficient did change after the introduction of presence into the model, indicating that presence and practice time covary, which is evidenced by the high correlation between presence and linear and quadratic play time ($r = 0.599$ and $r = 0.481$ respectively).

3.7. Hypothesis 3: Associations between Scores

We hypothesized that the AQ pre-test scores were significantly associated with VR anxiety ratings after the first session. Moreover, we hypothesized that the AQ pre-test scores would be significantly associated with a reduction in acrophobia symptoms, but not with VR exercise time. The results showed that the pre-test AQ scores were significantly associated with the subjective fear rating after the first session (r = 0.134, p <0.05) and a reduction in AQ scores at post-test (r = −0.312, $p < 0.05$). However, contrary to our hypothesis, AQ pre-test scores were not associated with either linear practice time (r = 0.006, p >0.05) or quadratic practice time (r = −0.003, $p > 0.05$).

3.8. Hypothesis 4: Repeated Activity in a VR Level Leads to a Consistent Decrease in Post-Level Anxiety

We hypothesized that, consistent with general expectations about exposure therapy, self-reported fear would show consistently lower scores after a session when compared to before a level, since repeated exposure should result in lower fear levels after a session. As can be seen in Table 3, this is the case for each level, with an average drop of 1.35 points (SD 2.24) per level. As seen in the minimum and maximum scores, some participants exit levels with higher fear ratings than they started with, indicating unsuccessful exposure exercises.

Table 3. Mean decrease in self-reported fear after completing each session.

Variable	N	Mean	SD	Min	Max
Level 1	4	−3.500	3.873	−9	0
Level 1–2	6	−0.833	2.562	−6	1
Level 1–3	6	−0.167	2.562	−4	4
Level 1–4	11	−1.545	2.911	−6	4
Level 1–5	39	−1.333	1.644	−6	0
TOTAL	66	−1.345	2.243	−9	4

4. Discussion

To our knowledge, this is the first study to look at self-guided VR exposure on a session-to-session basis. As self-guided exposure relies strongly on the participant to guide the progress through increasingly more challenging sessions, the inter-session data provides relevant information to guide future development of similar interventions. Moreover, successful exposure therapy relies on adequately modulating how challenging the different sessions are. This makes it important to verify that successful exposure took place within a session—as witnessed by a decreased anxiety level after a session as compared to before a session—in the absence of a therapist to guide this. Consistent with expectations from exposure therapy, the results indicate that overall, participants reported a decrease in fear as they progressed through the levels. It should be noted, however, that for some participants the exit scores remained relatively high, indicating unsuccessful exposure. The results further demonstrated that post-test AQ scores depended quadratically on time spent practicing, but not with the number of sessions practiced, indicating that it might be more important to play one level for a longer period of time instead of practicing many VR levels. Moreover, it was shown that, in line with previous research, a higher presence was associated with better outcomes [23].

Most participants advanced through all five of the VR exposure levels, indicating that—even in the absence of a therapist—self-guided VR therapy in the home setting is feasible and can be effective, even with rudimentary equipment such as a cardboard VR viewer and the participants' own smartphones. Importantly, the relatively high number of participants who completed all levels shows that the app was engaging and convincing enough to persuade participants to keep practicing. This motivational aspect is reflected by the number of sessions participants practiced, where on average participants tried each level at least twice, and in some cases up to 11 times. One explanation is that the threshold set for going to a subsequent level through levels (a self-reported fear of less than 4) added an element of challenge to the exposure, motivating participants to keep trying a level to unlock the next [34]. However, evidence for the success of gamification in smartphone apps is currently lacking [35].

Although existing VR interventions have been envisaged as solutions to be used in guided form under the supervision of a therapist (see e.g., [24]), ZeroPhobia was designed as a fully self-guided intervention with no therapist oversight. Therefore, it was crucial to monitor participant progression to verify whether successful in-virtuo exposure was taking place. When practicing with exposure exercises, it is important to correctly pace the increase in difficulty and challenge. Progressing too quickly through levels could result in excessive anxiety, leading to dropout, while practicing at an easy level for too long is inefficient and may lead the participant to disengage because it is not challenging enough. In ZeroPhobia it seems that these decisions were in line with the recommendations on pacing progress through the levels as shown in the app. In Table 2 it is shown that the average final anxiety scores in the levels were all below 4, since participants could not progress unless their self-reported fear had dropped under 4. This is visible in the self-reported fear levels after practicing a level for the first time. These averages also show that participants tended to 'level up', and not unhelpfully linger in levels. As most participants progressed to the highest level of the VR exposure game (level 5), it was not possible to find a reliable cut-off value for number of levels that should be completed, or to find a level that should minimally be attained for deriving clinical benefit; but the corollary is that participants chose to persist with the exposure exercises until the end, indicating successful and perhaps even enjoyable exposure experiences. However, we did find that increased activity was related to lower AQ scores at post-test. Results also demonstrated an association between decrease in AQ scores and practice time and number of sessions, suggesting the existence of a 'sweet spot', an optimum level of exposure at which increasing practice time does not result in increased benefit. In this study we found that participants derive most benefit when the practice time in the VR environment is 25.5 min irrespective of the amount of VR sessions. However, these results need to be interpreted with caution because it is unknown how many participants practiced for how long with the 360 videos.

The results showed that the pre-test AQ scores were significantly associated with the subjective fear rating after the first session and a reduction in AQ scores at post-test. This would suggest that those with higher acrophobia symptoms could derive more benefit from the VR exposure. This is also in line with previous research findings [11]. It could however also be a floor effect, where participants with already relatively low acrophobia symptoms have relatively little to gain from the intervention. Regardless, the results show that the VR environment offers a safe and engaging way to self-guided exposure, even for those with more severe complaints.

Limitations

The current study had several limitations. Firstly, all the hypotheses in this study were exploratory in nature, leading to the possibility of false positive findings. Secondly, more granular data in terms of logins and time spent in app modules would have been helpful for a more detailed view of user activity within the VR sessions. Thirdly, we did not have access to usage data of the 360 videos from YouTube. This means that several participants have practiced with 360° video exposure which could also contribute to a decrease in anxiety ratings at post-test. The optimum level of exposure time is a conservative estimate therefore. Fourthly, we did not systematically conduct data on the performance of the cardboard VR viewer during the sessions, therefore we are unable to evaluate the interaction of the performance of the VR viewer on its usage and effectiveness. However, only one participant contacted the research team to request a new viewer because the one originally provided to them had broken. Fifthly, due to a small sample size, some insignificant result may be the result of lack of statistical power. The great inter-subject variability in usage is remarkable. It might be that, depending on the personal history, VR stimulation will work at one moment of exposure, without a tool to identify the triggering event, conditioning success of fear reduction. Sixthly, data quality can be a problem in an uncontrolled environment, when only relying on self-report measures and no biological measures. However, research has demonstrated that self-report measures can have good to excellent validity when compared to a diagnostic interview [36]. Furthermore, participants can be more honest with filling in the questionnaires, as the computer has no 'eyebrows' [37]. Moreover, in a meta-analysis targeting VR interventions, Morina et al. [9] concluded that the behavioural measurement effect sizes were similar to those calculated from self-report measures in the VR studies, indicating no differences between the two types of measurements. Furthermore, we have conducted robustness analysis which confirmed that the VR-CBT ZeroPhobia app had a strong impact on the anxiety for heights, even when analyzed very conservatively in a randomized controlled design, and that the general anxiety effect did not drive the results. Lastly, as yet we have no data on external validity, especially on whether the effects of the VR exposure translate to decreased acrophobia and acrophobic avoidance in real-world settings, and commensurate increases in quality of life.

Future research is needed to replicate the main results of the study, especially with regard to external validity and translational effects in real life. Furthermore, more granular data on, e.g., eye gaze could generate valuable information on which cues participants choose to engage with, as even in VR participants can choose to look away from the fear-inducing stimulus. It would also be interesting to investigate whether adding sound to the VR experience effects the feeling of presence.

5. Conclusions

In sum, our findings show that self-guided VR for acrophobia symptoms is feasible, effective, and follows the same general patterns in terms of self-reported fear reductions as one would expect from therapist-guided exposure exercise. The results indicate that participants were engaged with ZeroPhobia as can be seen by the majority of them advancing through all VR exposure levels. Overall, fear levels decreased when participants progressed through the levels. Furthermore, our results suggest that it might be more beneficial to play one level for a longer period of time instead of practicing many VR levels and the existence of a 'sweet spot', an optimum level of exposure at which increasing practice time does not result in increased benefit. In this study we found that participants derive most benefit when the practice time in the VR environment is 25.5 min irrespective of the amount of VR sessions. Finally, the importance of feeling present in the VR environment is stressed out as a higher reported presence was associated with better outcomes. Further research is needed to see if the gains from VR translate into long-term sustained results, both in virtual and in real-life situations.

Supplementary Materials: The following are available online at http://www.mdpi.com/2077-0383/9/6/1614/s1, Figure S1: screenshots of ZeroPhobia; Figure S2: Variation in practicing duration for users who experienced at least one VR session.

Author Contributions: T.D. conceptualized the study, conceived the study, designed the study, contributed to survey design and data collection and wrote the manuscript. C.v.K. and I.C. performed the data analysis, wrote the method and result section and critically revised the manuscript. R.N.K. interpreted and drafted the results and discussion section and critically revised the manuscript. J.-L.v.G. contributed to the concept and design of the study and provided administrative, technical and material support and critically revised the manuscript. All authors contributed toward drafting and critically revising the paper, gave final approval of the version to be published, and agreed to be accountable for all aspects of the work. All authors have read and agreed to the published version of the manuscript.

Funding: This research was funded by NWO Toegepaste en Technische Wetenschappen (grant number 2016/STW/00099738), and NWO Creative Industrie-KIEM (grant number: 314-98-076).

Acknowledgments: The authors extend their gratitude to all the participants of the study, Bruno de Vos for designing ZeroPhobia, Doruk Eker for programming ZeroPhobia, Rufus van Baardwijk for ZeroPhobia sound, and Stefanie van Esveld and Niclas Fischer for assistance in data recruitment and data collection.

Conflicts of Interest: T.D. and J.-L.v.G. have developed the VR application ZeroPhobia which is used in the present study in collaboration with the Vrije Universiteit. ZeroPhobia is intended for commercial release. Hence, T.D. and J.-L.v.G. have not been involved in data analysis or any decisions related to the publication of findings. The other authors declare that they have no competing interests.

References

1. Donker, T.; Cornelisz, I.; van Klaveren, C.; van Straten, A.; Carlbring, P.; Cuijpers, P.; van Gelder, J.L. Effectiveness of self-guided app-based virtual reality cognitive behavior therapy for acrophobia: A randomized clinical trial. *JAMA Psychiatry* **2019**, *76*, 682–690. [CrossRef] [PubMed]
2. Fairburn, C.G.; Patel, V. The impact of digital technology on psychological treatments and their dissemination. *Behav. Res. Ther.* **2017**, *88*, 19–25. [CrossRef] [PubMed]
3. Andersson, G.; Carlbring, P.; Titov, N.; Lindefors, N. Internet interventions for adults with anxiety and mood disorders: A narrative umbrella review of recent meta-analyses. *Can. J. Psychiatry* **2019**. [CrossRef] [PubMed]
4. Andersson, G.; Cuijpers, P.; Carlbring, P.; Riper, H.; Hedman, E. Guided Internet-based vs. face-to-face cognitive behavior therapy for psychiatric and somatic disorders: A systematic review and meta-analysis. *World Psychiatry* **2014**, *13*, 288–295. [CrossRef] [PubMed]
5. Berger, T.; Boettcher, J.; Caspar, F. Internet-based guided self-help for several anxiety disorders: A randomized controlled trial comparing a tailored with a standardized disorder-specific approach. *Psychother. Chic.* **2014**, *51*, 207–219. [CrossRef] [PubMed]
6. Fodor, L.A.; Coteț, C.D.; Cuijpers, P.; Szamoskozi, S.; David, D.; Cristea, I.A. The effectiveness of virtual reality based interventions for symptoms of anxiety and depression: A meta-analysis. *Sci. Rep.* **2018**, *8*, 10323. [CrossRef] [PubMed]

7. Carl, E.; Stein, A.T.; Levihn-Coon, A.; Pogue, J.R.; Rothbaum, B.; Emmelkamp, P.; Asmundson, G.J.G.; Carlbring, P.; Powers, M.B. Virtual reality exposure therapy for anxiety and related disorders: A meta-analysis of randomized controlled trials. *J. Anxiety Disord.* **2019**, *61*, 27–36. [CrossRef]
8. Opris, D.; Pintea, S.; Garcia-Palacios, A.; Botella, C.; Szamoskozi, S.; David, D. Virtual reality exposure therapy in anxiety disorders: A quantitative meta-analysis. *Depress Anxiety* **2012**, *29*, 85–93. [CrossRef]
9. Morina, N.; Ijntema, H.; Meyerbröker, K.; Emmelkamp, P.M.G. Can virtual reality exposure therapy gains be generalized to real-life? A meta-analysis of studies applying behavioral assessments. *Behav. Res. Ther.* **2015**, *74*, 18–24. [CrossRef]
10. Parsons, T.D.; Rizzo, A.A. Affective outcomes of virtual reality exposure therapy for anxiety and specific phobias: A meta-analysis. *J. Behav. Ther. Exp. Psychiatry* **2008**, *39*, 250–261. [CrossRef]
11. Hong, Y.J.; Kim, H.E.; Jung, Y.H.; Kveong, S.; Kim, J.J. Usefulness of the mobile virtual reality self-training for overcoming a fear of heights. *Cyberpsychol. Behav. Soc. Netw.* **2017**, *20*, 753–761. [CrossRef] [PubMed]
12. van den Berg, S.W.; Peters, E.J.; Kraaijeveld, J.F.; Gielissen, M.F.; Prins, J.B. Usage of a generic web-based self-management intervention for breast cancer survivors: Substudy analysis of the BREATH trial. *J. Med. Internet Res.* **2013**, *15*, e170. [CrossRef] [PubMed]
13. Ritterband, L.M.; Thorndike, F.P.; Cox, D.J.; Kovatchev, B.P.; Gonder-Frederick, L.A. A behavior change model for internet interventions. *Ann. Behav. Med.* **2009**, *38*, 18–27. [CrossRef] [PubMed]
14. Sieverink, F.; Kelders, S.; Akkersdijk, S.; Poel, M.; Siemons, L.; van Gemert-Pijnen, L. Work in Progress: A Protocol for the Collection, Analysis, and Interpretation of Log Data from eHealth Technology. In Proceedings of the Fourth International Workshop on Behavior Change Support Systems (BCSS 2016), Salzburg, Austria, 5–7 April 2016; pp. 56–60.
15. Donkin, L.; Christensen, H.; Naismith, S.L.; Neal, B.; Hickie, I.B.; Glozier, N. A systematic review of the impact of adherence on the effectiveness of e-therapies. *J. Med. Internet Res.* **2011**, *13*, e52. [CrossRef]
16. Donkin, L.; Hickie, I.B.; Christensen, H.; Naismith, S.L.; Neal, B.; Cockayne, N.L.; Glozier, N. Rethinking the dose-response relationship between usage and outcome in an online intervention for depression: Randomized controlled trial. *J. Med. Internet. Res.* **2013**, *15*, e231. [CrossRef]
17. Van Gemert-Pijnen, J.E.; Kelders, S.M.; Bohlmeijer, E.T. Understanding the usage of content in a mental health intervention for depression: An analysis of log data. *J. Med. Internet. Res.* **2014**, *16*, e27. [CrossRef]
18. Manwaring, J.L.; Bryson, S.W.; Goldschmidt, A.B.; Winzelberg, A.J.; Luce, K.H.; Cunning, D.; Wilfley, D.E.; Taylor, C.B. Do adherence variables predict outcome in an online program for the prevention of eating disorders? *J. Consult. Clin. Psychol.* **2008**, *76*, 341–346. [CrossRef]
19. Cobb, N.K.; Graham, A.L.; Bock, B.C.; Papandonatos, G.; Abrams, D.B. Initial evaluation of a real-world internet smoking cessation system. *Nicotine Tob. Res.* **2005**, *7*, 207–216. [CrossRef]
20. Welding, K.; De Leon, E.; Cha, S.; Johnson, M.; Cohen, J.E.; Graham, A.L. Weekly enrollment and usage patterns in an Internet smoking cessation intervention. *Internet Interv.* **2017**, *9*, 100–105. [CrossRef]
21. Kelders, S.M.; Bohlmeijer, E.T.; Van Gemert-Pijnen, J.E. Participants, usage, and use patterns of a web-based intervention for the prevention of depression within a randomized controlled trial. *J. Med. Internet Res.* **2013**, *15*, e172. [CrossRef]
22. Bossen, D.; Buskermolen, M.; Veenhof, C.; de Bakker, D.; Dekker, J. Adherence to a web-based physical activity intervention for patients with knee and/or hip osteoarthritis: A mixed method study. *J. Med. Internet Res.* **2013**, *15*, e223. [CrossRef] [PubMed]
23. Gromer, D.; Reinke, M.; Christner, I.; Pauli, P. Causal interactive links between presence and fear in virtual reality height exposure. *Front. Psychol.* **2019**, *10*, 141. [CrossRef] [PubMed]
24. Wiederhold, B.K.; Bouchard, S. *Advances in Virtual Reality and Anxiety Disorders*; Springer: Boston, MA, USA, 2014; ISBN 978-1-4899-8022-9.
25. Lindner, P.; Miloff, A.; Hamilton, W.; Carlbring, P. The potential of consumer-targeted virtual reality relaxation applications: Descriptive usage, uptake and application performance statistics for a first-generation application. *Front. Psychol.* **2019**, *10*, 132. [CrossRef]
26. Beck, A.T.; Rush, A.J.; Shaw, B.F.; Emery, G. *Cognitive Therapy of Depression*; Guilford Press: New York, NY, USA, 1979.
27. Donker, T.; Van Esveld, S.; Fischer, N.; Van Straten, A. 0Phobia—Towards a virtual cure for acrophobia: Study protocol for a randomized controlled trial. *Trials* **2018**, *19*, 433. [CrossRef] [PubMed]

28. Cohen, D.C. Comparison of self-report and overt-behavioral procedures for assessing acrophobia. *Behav. Ther.* **1977**, *8*, 17–23. [CrossRef]
29. Steinman, S.A.; Teachman, B.A. Cognitive processing and acrophobia: Validating the Heights Interpretation Questionnaire. *J. Anxiety Disord.* **2011**, *25*, 896–902. [CrossRef]
30. Kroenke, K.; Spitzer, R.L.; Williams, J.B.W. The PHQ-9. *J. Gen. Intern. Med.* **2001**, *16*, 606–613. [CrossRef]
31. Donker, T.; van Straten, A.; Marks, I.M.; Cuijpers, P. A Brief web-based screening questionnaire for common mental disorders: Development and validation. *J. Med. Internet Res.* **2009**, *11*, e19. [CrossRef]
32. Survalyzer Nederland, B.V. Home. Available online: https://www.survalyzer.com/ (accessed on 2 July 2019).
33. Schubert, T.; Friedmann, F.; Regenbrecht, H. The experience of presence: Factor analytic insights. *Presence Teleoper. Virtual Environ.* **2001**, *10*, 266–281. [CrossRef]
34. King, D.; Greaves, F.; Exeter, C.; Darzi, A. "Gamification": Influencing health behaviours with games. *J. R. Soc. Med.* **2013**, *106*, 76–78. [CrossRef]
35. Edwards, E.A.; Lumsden, J.; Rivas, C.; Steed, L.; Edwards, L.A.; Thiyagarajan, A.; Sohanpal, R.; Caton, H.; Griffiths, C.J.; Munafò, M.R.; et al. Gamification for health promotion: Systematic review of behaviour change techniques in smartphone apps. *BMJ Open* **2016**, *6*, e012447. [CrossRef] [PubMed]
36. Evans, M.; Kessler, D.; Lewis, G.; Peters, T.J.; Sharp, D. Assessing mental health in primary care research using standardized scales: Can it be carried out over the telephone? *Psychol. Med.* **2004**, *23*, 157–162. [CrossRef] [PubMed]
37. Marks, I.M.; Cavanagh, K.; Gega, L. Computer-aided psychotherapy: Revolution or bubble? *Br. J. Psychiatry* **2007**, *191*, 471–473. [CrossRef] [PubMed]

MDPI
St. Alban-Anlage 66
4052 Basel
Switzerland
Tel. +41 61 683 77 34
Fax +41 61 302 89 18
www.mdpi.com

Journal of Clinical Medicine Editorial Office
E-mail: jcm@mdpi.com
www.mdpi.com/journal/jcm

www.ingramcontent.com/pod-product-compliance
Lightning Source LLC
Chambersburg PA
CBHW041952260926
51850CB00019B/2674
9783039437351